Dedicated to all of those who

You are enough.

Table of Contents

Courage: n. "strength in the face of pain or grief."[1]

All of us are dealing with something in our lives that is painful or difficult and, because of these struggles, we are discovering who we are. Our struggles and experiences teach us new things and help to define us.

This may be depression, anxiety, an abusive relationship, an illness, losing a job, trying to find a way to pay this month's rent, etc. Whatever your struggles are, you are not alone. These struggles that we all face is called "life" and we deal with versions of them every day. However, it's how we deal with these struggles that matter the most.

As Mark Twain once said, "Courage is not the absence of fear; it is acting in spite of it."

For me, vaginismus is my struggle, and I have to learn how to show strength and courage every day so that I don't let it defeat me. Depression is constantly trying to bring me down, but I must learn to rise above that and not let it shackle me.

If you take anything away from this book, it is to not be so hard on yourself. You were given these struggles because you have the courage to overcome them.

Chapter 1: Sit Back and Enjoy the Journey...

As I mentioned in my blog, *Girl with the Paw Print Tattoo*, the first place that I truly opened up about my condition, I invite you

---

[1] Merriam-Webster Dictionary online, *"courage,"* 2018, np.

to grab a cup of coffee or tea and cuddle up in a nice warm blanket. We will delve into the purpose of this book and meet one another on a more personal level.

If you picked up this book, you might be suffering from the same, or a similar, condition. You might even be a concerned partner, who really wants to learn more about what your significant other is going through. Perhaps, you are even a doctor, looking to hear the perspective of a patient. Whatever brought you to this book, I hope you enjoy the ride and discover innovative ideas and thoughts.

Picture this, you are enjoying a romantic dinner with a new boyfriend, your fiancé, or husband. The table is set for two. Wine glasses are twinkling next to the light of the candles and the two of you laugh and smile at one another. After dinner, you head over to the couch to watch a movie. Of course, you are curious about the movie but, let's be honest, you are more interested in the person sitting next to you. He grabs your hand and you both turn to look at one another. Both of you lean forward as your lips touch. It doesn't take too long before both of you want to take this romantic moment to the bedroom. However, you can't. Not because you don't want to, but because you have dyspareunia. Your pubococcygeus (PC) muscles are telling you "No" when your body is saying, "Yes, I want to!"

Defeat, humiliation, embarrassment, sadness and guilt flood your thoughts. He looks at you with those sad, but understanding eyes, as you separate and continue watching the movie. All the while, your own eyes are welling up with tears and you can no longer concentrate on the romantic evening.

This is just one scenario that many women, who have vaginal pain, struggle with daily. However, very few talk about it to others because it seems like a strange, maybe even taboo, topic to discuss. Let's change that. Let's make sure that women, from all over the world and all walks of life, can open up and share their stories with the public. Sexual dysfunction among women is not a laughing matter, nor should it be an awkward discussion. Let's share our stories, so that more women feel free to open up and share theirs. You are not alone.

Vaginismus is just one pelvic pain condition that effects women of all ages and backgrounds. It does not discriminate and is kind to no one. There are two main types of vaginismus, each with a varying degree of pain. Primary vaginismus is where the woman has never experienced pain-free sex or penetration before. Secondary vaginismus is where the woman has once been able to experience pain-free sex, but something caused her to develop it later in life.

Vaginismus is where the PC muscles tense up, and this can be due to a variety of reasons. Past sexual trauma, a strict religious upbringing or even being highly sensitive and anxious are just a few of the common reasons.

Unfortunately, for those of us suffering with this condition, there are not many books out in the world that talk about vaginismus. Therefore, I began my blog to help women, who like myself, walk through this journey together. I have turned some of its passages into this book.

There are bound to be rough days, since vaginismus affects women physically and psychologically. However, we will get through them together. Anxiety and depression walk hand in hand with vaginismus and I would like to promote a positive atmosphere for all the women out there who are seeking advice or someone to talk to.

Just remember, you are enough!

Chapter 2: Signs & Symptoms

I had absolutely no clue what vaginismus was until I began dealing with the condition first hand. Even in the beginning, I was in denial that anything was wrong with me. I simply thought that sex hurt the first time you had it and that I just needed to learn to deal with it.

How many of you also pretended that painful sex was normal? How many of you were told that sex would be painful your first time? How many of you remained in denial after you had been diagnosed?

I answered "Yes" to all of these questions, and I know many of you did the same. It's common for women in our culture to be taught that sex is simply painful the first time you have it. Why is that? Most of the girls I know said it didn't hurt when they lost their virginity. So, what's with the lies? It could be a way to instill fear, so that girls don't experience sex too early in life. It could also be that some women do experience discomfort, which can be misconstrued as "pain," especially if that word has been schooled into their brains throughout their life. I mean, even the TV shows and movies bring it up!

In my youth, I was told that sex was dirty, and one needed to wait until marriage to have it, thanks to my religious upbringing and schooling. However, those are not the only factors relating to my vaginismus. It's a much more complicated condition than that.

After becoming more concerned with the pain that I was feeling after sex, I did a brief Google search and discovered that this pain was called "vaginismus." Because I didn't want my parents to know I was having sex, I pretended that I didn't have this problem and silently kept it to myself for months. It wasn't until I was in a session with my therapist that the pain was brought up and she helped me to seek real medical attention.

Now, not every doctor in my story plays a promising lead role. Some of my doctors turned out to be extremely incompetent. My first gynecologist knew I struggled with pain during examinations, yet never addressed it. Now, when I say "struggled," I mean I was literally held down on the table by two nurses as I cried and shook uncontrollably whenever she examined me. Half of the time she couldn't even examine me because my PC muscles blocked her. Yet, she still never addressed that there was a problem until I approached her saying that I believe I have this condition. Her response was, "Oh that makes sense! I always just thought you never liked exams."

Let's just take a moment of silence as we contemplate her ignorance.

Once officially diagnosed, I began to look for more information on my condition. I found that the definition was a, "Vaginal tightness causing discomfort, burning, pain, penetration problems, or complete inability to have intercourse. The vaginal tightness results from the involuntary tightening of the pelvic floor, especially the pubococcygeus (PC) muscle group..."[2]

The Diagnostic and Statistical Manual of Mental Disorders defines vaginismus as a "Genito-pelvic pain/penetration disorder."[3] This is where a woman is unable to achieve vaginal penetration despite the desire to do so. This can be with tampons, dilators, sex, examinations, etc.

So those are the medical definitions, but for those of us who enjoy a more creative description, I'll talk about that now...

Vaginismus is a real pain that can occur from either physical or non-physical events. For instance, physical pains that can trigger vaginismus are traumatic childbirth, surgeries, physical abuse and even illnesses or medical conditions that deal with the pelvic region. Non-physical causes can be a strict religious or non-religious upbringing, emotional abuse and anxiety or fears relating to sex. Women can suffer from one or multiple triggers.

---

[2] Mark and Lisa Carter, *Completely Overcome Vaginismus: The Practical Approach to Pain-Free Intercourse*, 2011, 19.
[3] *Diagnostic and Statistical Manual of Mental Disorders*, American Psychiatric Association, 5th, ed. 2013, np.

For people like myself, I suffer from non-physical triggers. Physically, nothing is wrong with me, but psychologically, I have undergone quite a bit of trauma and it is causing my PC muscles to go into self-defense mode, even if I don't want them to. Basically, I have had this problem for so long now (eight years, at the time of writing this) that it's second nature for my muscles to spasm without me even realizing it. The PC muscles believe that they are doing this to protect me, especially during sex or intimacy. Even intimacy like kissing, foreplay, hand holding, hugging and cuddling, cause me anxiety and my muscles tense up or spasm.

Pain can vary depending on the individual, and both Mark and Lisa Carter's book, *Completely Overcome Vaginismus*, and Peter T. Pacik's medical journal, *Understanding and treating vaginismus: a multimodal approach*, explain classifications of pain. Dr. Pacik was the first doctor to develop the Botox procedure for vaginismus. He states that there are 5 grades of pain during an examination and pain during penetration is scored 1-10, with 10 being the worst. Below, I have listed his 5 grades of pain during examinations:

> *Lamont grade 1: "Patient is able to relax for pelvic examination."*
> *Lamont grade 2: "Patient is unable to relax for pelvic examination."*
> *Lamont grade 3: "Buttocks lift off table. Early retreat."*
> *Lamont grade 4: "Generalized retreat: buttocks lift up, thighs close, patient retreats."*

*Pacik grade 5: "Generalized retreat as in level 4 plus
visceral reaction, which may result in any one or more of the
following: palpitations, hyperventilation, sweating, severe
trembling, uncontrollable shaking, screaming, hysteria, wanting to
jump off the table, a feeling of becoming unconscious, nausea,
vomiting, and even a desire to attack the doctor."[4]*

These medical pain spectrums can be helpful to understand where you lie on the spectrum, but when I am personally asked how it feels to have sex, I give them the "Are you ready?" look.

For me, it feels like you are being ripped apart. There is a burning sensation in the vagina and it feels like sandpaper is scraping against the layers of your vaginal wall. My personal favorite description for people, is that it feels like a metal shard is tearing away the inside of your vagina. It's unbearable and excruciating, so obviously your brain is going to react to this pain by tensing the muscles, so that nothing can get through.

Even though what I describe sounds extreme, I have had about seven different doctors and three physical therapists examine me to make sure nothing was wrong with me anatomically. Every time, the doctors were baffled because I looked healthy. Some would be kind and cry as they realized that they didn't know how to help me. Others would give advice or tell me to try harder to relax.

---

[4] Peter T. Pacik, *Understanding and treating vaginismus: a multimodal approach,* The International Urogynecology Association, 2014, 3.

However, in the next chapter, I will discuss various treatments that are out there and what I have personally tried.

Chapter 3: Treatments

I have already listed "Signs and Symptoms" in the previous chapter, but now I'm going to delve into various treatments that doctors have tried on individuals with vaginismus. This chapter is a list of treatment options that I have also personally experienced. Now, some women were able to overcome their vaginismus with only one type of treatment, some had to use a variety of treatments at once, but many ladies were unable to overcome vaginismus with any of these. Since there is an interplay of emotional and physical aspects of vaginismus, it can be hard to link one treatment for every woman.

Dilator treatment: Dilators come in various shapes and sizes. I was given the pediatric sizes and the vaginal dilators by a gynecologist. At first, I was simply given the boxes and not instructed on how to use them. It wasn't until six years into vaginismus that a physical therapist told me how to use them properly. This is not an uncommon problem for women.

The dilator is meant to help the individual overcome the physical and psychological aspects of vaginismus. You start with a small dilator in the beginning and work towards a larger size when you are ready. This slow progression should exercise the muscles, much like practicing to exercise for a marathon. I had been told by my physical therapist to use them for 10 to 15 minutes a day, along with exercises she gave me. Just recently, I was told by my therapist and psychiatrist to use them whenever I can and to use them whenever my fiancé and I got intimate, whether that means during massages or cuddling.

The unfortunate thing is that in my personal experience I become extremely depressed and cry uncontrollably. It comes to a point where I need to call someone to talk to because I feel like I should not be alone when dealing with that level of depression. Setting candles, burning incense, turning the lights off and putting music on all sound great in theory, but the reality is it is painfully depressing to use them, especially when I'm not gaining any progress after all these years.

Physical therapy: Physical therapists can greatly help with vaginismus if they are trained in dealing with pelvic floor disorders or pelvic pain. I have been to three physical therapists within two years. The first one I went to was wonderful and had me insert the dilators in her office, so that I was in a safe place while using them. She gave me biofeedback, had me wear electric shock pads for weeks to a month to relax the muscles, and even provided me with a variety of exercises and stretches that I still use today. Because of my aversion to touch, she would spend 10 to 15 minutes each session massaging my PC muscles and the sphincter muscles, while she counseled me. That combination was great, and I experienced results from her various combination of treatments. Believe it or not, I was able to experience a vaginal orgasm for the first time in my whole life.

Unfortunately, after a certain point, there was no more that could be done in her office and my insurance was no longer able to cover the appointments. I was sent home with worksheets, stretches and instructions to use the dilators daily. I was able to accomplish these exercises on my own for a month before the PC muscles began to tense again and I regressed.

The other two physical therapists that I saw are not particularly noteworthy to mention. They did not help much, and it became more of a burden to see them. I no longer see a physical therapist because the one I was seeing, who was supposedly the best in my town, said she didn't know how else to help me. I hear that a lot…

Counseling and therapy: Therapy has been helpful to me for many reasons. It has helped with the anxiety, depression and coming to terms with why I have vaginismus. Unfortunately, I still have my bad days. The use of Cognitive Behavioral Therapy is great for understanding the thoughts and feelings that have influenced vaginismus. LENS treatment is another form of treatment that I was given to help with anxiety and depression. Sensors are placed in specific areas on the "scalp to listen in on brainwave activity." These sessions are extremely brief, lasting a few minutes or less. [5]

My therapist is also communicating with a sex therapist, and we have recently developed a strategy that I am excited about. Exposure therapy. This is where I will gradually try simple intimacy

---

[5] "What is Neurofeedback?" OchsLabs: The Neurofeedback Experts, 2018, np.

exercises before leading up to anything major. For instance, I will work on receiving compliments first, since I've always been anxious when this would happen. Then, my fiancé and I will massage with our clothes on and eventually work to remove articles of clothing later on. Eventually, we will try kissing and if anxiety does come up, I acknowledge it's there but keep going. Without going any further into detail, you can kind of see the slow process and how it should lessen my anxiety down the road.

Hypnotherapy: I think this has always been a fun idea to me and, while I do become relaxed during a session, I have never been able to become so relaxed that the muscles stop spasming. However, I have been told by my psychiatrist that this method has worked for many.

Medication: I am currently taking four different types of medication. Anti-anxiety and anti-depressants. Both have helped tremendously with my anxiety and depression, but my psychiatrist and I are still working to find a nice balance that might ease the tension I feel with intimacy and sex.

Acupuncture: For about two years, I tried getting into taking herbal medications and really understanding homeopathic medicine. Unfortunately for me, it never worked. I felt like I was delving into the realm of the placebo effect and not gaining results. While the first acupuncturist I visited was very good and had me feeling relaxed, the effects were not long term.

Lidocaine: I was given lidocaine for about two years. While it helped with the dilators, it never worked during sex. It was more of a mask, simply hiding the actual problem I was dealing with and never turning around to face it.

Estrogen cream: This one did not work for me at all. In fact, it caused me to start bleeding vaginally and I was taken off of it immediately, so as not to cause me long term damage.

Botox: This is one that I have never tried and have been curious about. Some doctors have warned me about it; however, many women have said it was useful. At first, I was not entirely sure how this was used, but after some research, I discovered that vaginal injections are given to the patient until they are able to fully relax. I will talk about the Botox Treatment in depth in Chapters 7 and 8.

Other Treatments: I'm sure there are more treatments out there, but these are ones I am familiar with. I have also heard of CBD oil being used to help relax the muscles; however, I have not tried this for myself.

Chapter 4: Physical Therapy stretches for vaginismus

Physical therapy is one of the treatments to aid vaginismus. I had a wonderful physical therapist for a year, until my insurance stopped covering it and she reached a peak in her repertoire. During my time with her, I was able to have sex that wasn't as painful as before. It was one of the happiest moments in my life.

She spent an hour with me each day, having me insert the dilators, massaging the PC and rectal muscles, and having me do some breathing exercises. She even had me wear electric shock pads for months, having me increase the voltage every so often. It was designed to relax the muscles.

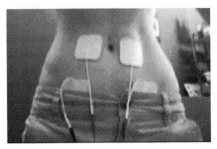

Every once and awhile, she would provide me with new stretches to relax the PC muscles. My favorite was **"The Drop,"** designed to work the opposite of a Kegel exercise. Instead of holding the muscles in, you relax them. The best way to describe it is to pretend like you are about to pee. That relaxation of the muscle is something you try to do throughout the day.

Below are pictures and descriptions of the various exercises she gave me written in my own words. I hope these help you, but please remember to be safe when performing them. If you feel like you are pushing yourself too much on the stretch, then stop and relax. We don't want any injuries here.

Diaphragmatic Breathing is one exercise that I will also mention in Chapter 5. My PT had me perform this exercise lying back, sitting and standing. However, when first performing this exercise, it is easier to do so lying down. Place one hand on your chest cavity and the other on your stomach. Make sure you are fully relaxed. When you inhale through your nose, let your stomach rise. Exhale through your mouse and let your stomach fall. She had me perform this exercise throughout the day.

Diaphragmatic Breathing with Movement is another great exercise that uses your pelvic floor muscles. Lay on your back and remain relaxed. When you inhale using the Diaphragmatic Breathing technique, move your feet out, and when you exhale, move your feet in. She had me perform 10 in the morning and 10 at night.

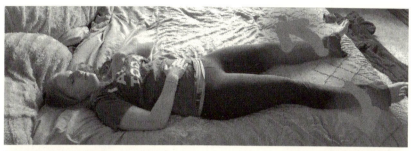

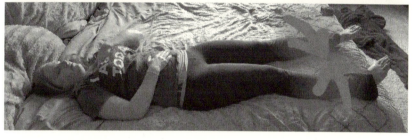

Incorporating diaphragmatic breathing with movement

Thigh Press is a very simple stretch that will relax the pelvic floor muscles. Lay on your back, put your knees up and place your hands on the outside of your knees. You want to push on your knees while your knees are pushing back. Hold this pose for five seconds and then relax. I was told to repeat this exercise five times twice a day.

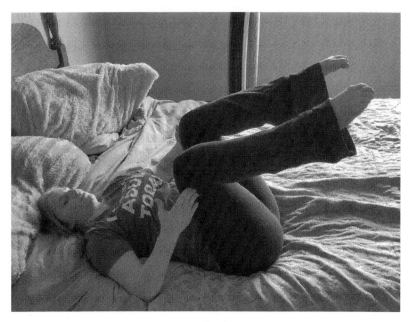

Thigh press

The Pelvic Floor Stretch is a lot like a wall sit or squat. You stand with your legs apart, keeping your back straight and squat down. Do three repetitions of this stretch twice a day for 30 to 60 seconds.

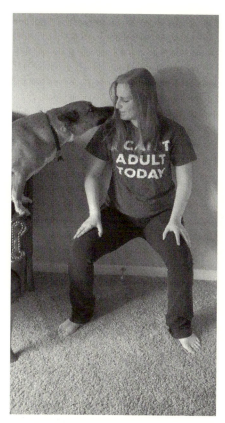

Pelvic floor stretch

You can also do this stretch while lying down.

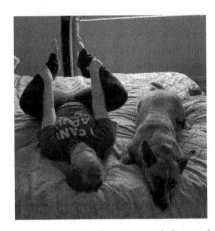

Example of pelvic floor stretch lying down

The Inner Thigh Stretches below are really helpful for your inner thigh close to the PC muscles. All three stretches are performed 5 times for 15 seconds daily.

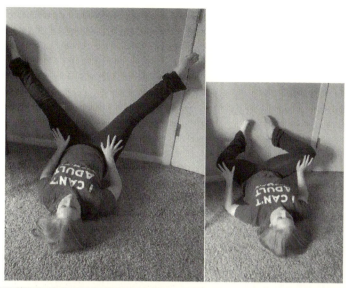

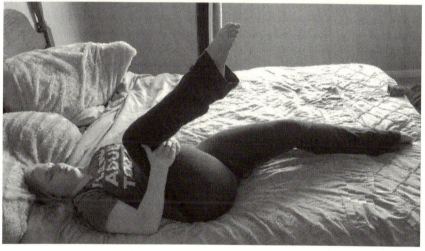

Chapter 5: Breathing Techniques

If you suffer from depression, anxiety or even just the everyday stresses of life, you can benefit from these five simple breathing techniques. There are many out there, but I'm going to list a few that have worked for me.

4-7-8 breathing technique: My therapist gave me this one when I first visited her. It's probably one of my favorites. Inhale through your nose while you count to four. Hold your breath to the count of seven. Exhale through your mouth for the count of eight.

Grounding: Another technique I enjoy is more of a grounding exercise. You want to sit in a chair and breathe quietly through your nose and out through your mouth. As you do that, think of yourself sinking deeper and deeper into the chair. Let yourself fall into it. Relax your face, your toes, your fingers, your legs and arms. Think of nothing but sinking into your seat, as though you are deepening yourself into the soil, growing roots and becoming a sturdy tree.

Three Part Breathing: I learned this next exercise in a yoga class, and it has helped me with anxiety. It is often used during Savasana. You lay on your back with your arms by your side. You relax every muscle in your face and in your body. You can even turn on calming music if that helps you to relax. Make sure that, even though you are focusing on relaxing every muscle, you are also breathing. The breaths you take are quiet and deep. You want to start by placing your hand on your upper chest. Inhale into your chest, through the upper part of your abdomen, and finally through your belly so that it puffs out. Slowly release your breath in and exhale through the belly, then through your upper abdomen and finally through your chest.

Diaphragmatic Breathing: This is another technique that was given to me in physical therapy and helps those with pelvic pain. You want to lay on your back in a bed with your legs out. Place one hand on your chest and the other on your stomach. When you inhale, let your abdomen rise. When you exhale, let your abdomen fall. You want to make sure you are not breathing through your chest. Your hand on your chest should be steady, while the one on your stomach is moving with each breath.

Calming your mood: The last one helps if you are needing to calm your thoughts or your mood. You sit on a chair and bend forward so that your head is almost touching the floor. Let your arms fall. Let your body relax and sink. Sit there for a few moments and breathe quietly in through your nose and exhale through your mouth. Do this until you feel a sense of calm.

Other Techniques and Exercises: Feel free to light incense or a candle. Perhaps even turning off or dimming the lights while you do these breathing techniques will help calm your mind. Personally, listening to nature sounds, meditation music or frequency music helps me. Although, I know many prefer the silence.

Guided meditation narratives are also extremely helpful. Sometimes, it's difficult to calm your mind on your own, but having someone guide you through the meditation dissipates your everyday thoughts because you are simply focusing on their voice.

If you are unable to find a guided meditation narrative, you can also discover your mantra. A mantra is a word or phrase that you say repeatedly to keep the mind focused and engaged. A mantra can be anything like, "This shall pass," "I choose happiness," or "Breathe in calm. Breathe out anxiety." Personalize your mantra depending on what positive energy you would like to release. A mantra is meant to help you heal, become a stronger person or calm and focus your mind.

I hope one of these helps you!

Chapter 6: Exposure Therapy for Vaginismus

What exactly is Exposure Therapy? Exposure therapy is a type of cognitive-behavioral therapy that can help individuals overcome their fears and anxieties. This is done by gradually exposing the patient to the source of their anxiety in hopes that they will overcome their fear and live normal lives.

How does this form of therapy help people who have vaginismus? Vaginismus is caused by anxiety, fears or even traumatic events. Exposure therapy is all about creating a safe place for that person, so that they can control their anxiety. My therapist and a sex therapist are using this therapy technique to help me become less anxious around intimacy. Without delving right into sex, they are having me gradually expose myself to various types of intimacy. They also provided me with a book titled, *For Yourself: The Fulfillment of Female Sexuality*, by Lonnie Garfield Barbach. Unfortunately, I had to stop reading the book because the women in the book were simply there to experience an orgasm, not to deal with painful sex. It made me feel quite upset and I couldn't understand how this book was designed to help me. Now, I see that it's meant to show me that I shouldn't be afraid of sexuality. It's completely normal and not dirty at all, unlike my religious upbringing taught me. Nevertheless, due to my reaction, my therapist suggested I put down the book until I am ready to pick it up again.

A few stages of exposure therapy, when dealing with vaginismus, might go something like this:

First, I would be rubbing my hands and arms to understand the feel of touch. However, I would be in control. Through this technique, I will also learn what type of touch I enjoy.

Second, would be to have my fiancé give me a massage and I give him one.

Third, would be to kiss and cuddle.

Fourth, would be to become comfortable being around him without clothes on.

Fifth, would be cuddling, kissing or massaging with a dilator inserted, and so on and so forth…

I think you can understand that after taking little steps like this for months, maybe even a year, I should be able to become less anxious when any form of sex or serious intimacy occurs.

I am excited to try this method and I truly think it will help ease my mind and fears whenever I think about sex. Normally, I dread or avoid any intimacy whatsoever, but I feel that, with this gradual exposure in a safe environment, I will be able to break that cycle of distress. I will admit that it has been difficult for me to keep up with the therapy daily. Some days, I just prefer to be alone and want my own space, while other days I am okay with cuddling and enjoying each other's company. However, I am not to the point yet where I can insert the dilators during cuddling or massaging because I can't find the motivation to use them. For me, they are a pain to insert and often cause me to become more depressed.

I believe that this form of therapy can also be applied to others fears as well, but always be sure to consult with a professional beforehand.

Chapter 7: Botox Treatment

When I had done research on Botox, it had been years ago. I gained a great deal of my information from women on a forum at www.vaginismus.com. I heard stories about how it is dangerous and how not much is known about it. I completely ruled it out for myself, until recently.

My fiancé and I were sitting on the couch enjoying a movie when I brought up Botox. He said he hadn't heard me mention that form of treatment before. I told him I stopped looking into it after I heard some extreme stories and figured I would just be putting poison into my body. I mean thinking about it, getting Botox injections in your vaginal muscles does sound terrifying. We view Botox as a toxin because the drug is made from botulinum toxin type A, so why would you want it near that delicate area? However, since that night, we have both been doing more research on it and discovered some interesting cases which I will share with you now.

Vaginismus MD – On this website, it states that a small dosage of Botox, 100 to 150 units, is inserted into the three important muscles in the vagina. Even though Botox usually only lasts for four to six months, by that time, the patient will have achieved pain free sex and their brain will no longer fear sex or intimacy. The brain will send positive signals to the muscles to stop them from spasming, even after the injections wear off, because you would have experienced only comfortable and painless sex. The results of the injections are supposed to be immediate, between two to five days. There are minor risks, like incontinence.[6]

One Girl's Success Story – This is a story about a young girl, who managed to achieve pain free sex after having Botox injections. For six years, she struggled to have sex, and doctors were constantly looking to pinpoint a trigger. She was told to try various treatments, like yoga, meditation and dilators, and doctors also found nothing to be wrong with her physically (sounds familiar!) Eventually, after reading the book, *When Sex Seems Impossible*, that described Botox treatment for vaginismus, she decided to investigate receiving them. They are expensive and most insurance companies do not cover them. Since vaginismus is mostly a mental block, some insurance companies are not going to pay for something that is not physically wrong with you. Most insurance companies will also not cover claims that are not deemed detrimental to your health. Vaginal pain is not considered detrimental to your health and, as far as they see it, is not going to

---

[6] Peter T. Pacik, Vaginismus MD, *How, Why and How Often is Botox Used to Treat Vaginismus?* 2018, np.

cause you any serious problems in the future. Nevertheless, she managed to get the money and had the procedure done. Two weeks later, she was having pain free sex with her boyfriend.[7]

2014 Case Report – Remember our good friend Dr. Pacik? Well, he is making an appearance once again! He is the doctor that developed this procedure to treat vaginismus. This case report talks about a 28-year-old woman, who was diagnosed with vaginismus and was unable to achieve pain free sex with her husband of one year. After receiving the procedure, she was successfully able to have pain free sex with him 10 days afterwards. They point out that this procedure is not a cure for vaginismus, but an aid. They state the procedure, coupled with therapy and dilator use, can help a patient overcome vaginismus for good.[8]

Botox Changed My Life – A woman named Lara received Botox injections and was astounded by the results. Even though she still has to put a lot of work into tackling the condition, since she has more than just vaginismus, she said the procedure has made things a bit easier. She still must use the dilators and her stretches daily, but she can see the dramatic difference from before and after. For her, sexual intercourse still isn't easy, but due to the progression she is making, she feels that it will happen in her near future. Again,

---

[7] Catriona Harvey-Jenner, "I had to have botox in my vagina so I could lose my virginity," Cosmopolitan, April 10, 2017, np.

[8] Werner MA, Pacik PT, Ferrara M, Marcus BS, *Botox for the Treatment of Vaginismus: A Case Report*, Journal of Women's Health Care, 2014, np.

she does state that this was not a cure-all for her and she also mentions that the procedure is not cheap.[9]

With continued efforts to get information out there about vaginismus, we all hope that more research will go into finding a better treatment or cure for those of us who struggle with the condition.

The last report is a **Clinical Trial**, where 31 participants, between the ages of 20 to 37, were given 150 units of Botox injections. All the participants were analyzed and 90.3% were able to achieve pain free intercourse. Zero percent of the participants experienced any adverse effects. In one year, the patients were re-evaluated and were still able to have pain free sex. This clinical trial was also performed by Dr. Pacik.[10]

There are a few additional stories out there explaining the same things, but feel free to read them on your own time if you need to. However, the three takeaways that we can gather from all the stories up above are:

It is expensive. Not every insurance will cover a procedure like this. Many have stated it is not a cure-all if you have more than vaginismus. Sometimes, as with many surgeries, work is still needed to be done after the procedure. It has an 80-90% success rate for women, who have vaginismus, to experience pain free sex or at least a jump start in using dilators.

---

[9] Devin Lytle, "I Got Botox In My Vagina And It Changed My Life," BuzzFeed, January 13, 2017, np.
[10] Peter T. Pacik, "Botox Injection for Treatment of Vaginismus," U.S. National Library of Medicine, 2017, np.

Another concern of mine is finding a place, either in my city or close by, that performs this delicate procedure and performs it well. I am willing to try it but know it won't be for a while. I feel a little bit of hope with this discovery, so I wanted to share it with you. If you are looking into it as well be sure to do your own research or, if are reading about it for the first time, I hope that you learned something interesting today.

Chapter 8: Botox stories from women

I started watching a TV show on Netflix called *Embarrassing Bodies*, and immediately clicked on the vagina episode. Yes, that's my life now. I was desperately hoping I'd find someone in the episode, who struggled with vaginismus.

Well, sadly, I did not encounter anyone. However, one person did have to get Botox injections for a different problem (her muscles were not tightening after childbirth).

When I watched the procedure, I became a little uneasy. It is quite invasive and scary looking, especially for someone who hates needles. Nevertheless, despite the medical journals I uncovered, I decided that I wanted to interview real women, who have experienced Botox, to help ease my mind.

What I discovered was that not a lot of women are available to discuss their Botox procedure. This could be due to the fact that not many women have undergone the surgery. Unfortunately, I was unable to get interviews as easily as I had in Chapter 12.

There are many stories of women, who have experienced or undergone the Botox procedure on Reddit; however, I never received permission by all of the ladies to use their stories. I can tell you that there were mixed reactions to receiving the Botox procedure. Some of the women said it helped with their dilator progression, while others said that it didn't help them to gain any headway. One thing that all of them could agree on was that it was extremely expensive and most insurance companies do not cover it as was mentioned in Chapter 7. The other information I gathered was that some of them had anesthesia but others didn't. The ones who didn't said that it was a very painful procedure and felt like a pop in your muscles. Take note ladies and get the drugs!

From the women who did contact me back, one explained that, prior to Botox, she had been struggling to insert the largest dilator. She had been working on using the dilators on and off again up until the months following her procedure. She had been put under anesthesia during the procedure and felt no pain afterwards. She woke up with the largest dilator inserted. She was told to keep it inserted for 24 hours and had a variety of dilator work that needed to be done after she received her injections. One important thing to note is that her doctor mentioned that many women who don't use the dilators following their procedure do not have the same positive results.

Another woman, named Eilis, explained that, while Botox did help her insert the dilators, pain was still there. She said it's not a cure-all and she still has to go back to get her injections redone. For her, it wasn't a onetime treatment. She also explained that after the procedure she had horrible cramps and bruising, which I pretty much expected. Here is a little snippet of her experience:

"The top layer of my vaginal skin was numbed, but the 'pop' into the muscle was entirely something I could feel…For that, I wished I was under."

She went on to explain that the experience was like having a trigger point in your vagina and someone pressing on it but going through layers and layers of deep tissue. Pleasant. She also explained it didn't help her to overcome the emotional trauma she had that triggers her vaginismus.

The last lady I interviewed, who struggles with endometriosis, stated that she noticed a regression after her Botox wore off. She said,

"Before Botox, I couldn't insert anything at all and all the muscles in my pelvic floor were like concrete. Now the Botox has worn off I've noticed that I'm struggling to insert the second dilator whereas before I could insert it without pain." However, she has recently received her second set of injections and noticed that she was able to insert a tampon now.

One woman on Reddit, Caitlin, responded to her by saying that, "This is the exact reason my PT doesn't recommend Botox. It's a temporary fix."

Overall, from what I gathered through these experiences, Botox is a great starting point for you. However, it is not a "cure-all." Some women have had wonderful experiences and do swear by this procedure, but not everybody is the same. It also sounds like something that requires additional time and effort from your part, whether that is through therapy or the dilators. It's one of those things that you have to decide if the risk is worth the cost. Will you spend the ridiculous amount of money for the procedure to see if it will work for you, or will you not do it and spend your years wondering, "what if?"

Chapter 9: Pelvic Health Support and Summit

Many women out there silently suffer from pelvic pain and bringing awareness to it will certainly make those women more comfortable with seeking help. I was extremely cautious and nervous to mention to anyone that I have vaginismus. I saw it as a condition that would be laughed at or even made a taboo topic. However, pelvic pain is real, and thousands of women suffer from it in varying degrees.

In addition to this, those of you who suffer from pelvic pain, like vaginismus, endometriosis, or vulvodynia, I have another resource for you that may be helpful. I stumbled upon this site when I was looking for more information on vaginismus. This website provides quality content and support based on your interests and/or conditions. They also have a Facebook group, which I have joined. The organization is Pelvic Health Support and, if you are interested, register for free and request to join their Facebook group.

This group looks at all different types of pelvic pain, and even IBS, which I also suffer from. They discuss both holistic and modern medicine, instead of leaning on one over the other. I like this approach best because sometimes things happen that science just can't explain.

During the month of May, which is Pelvic Health Awareness Month, the group had a Pelvic Health Summit, where various pelvic health professionals were interviewed.

Amy Stein's interview

The interview that struck me the most was one with Amy Stein, a pelvic floor physical therapist and past president of the International Pelvic Pain Society. She spoke "about the awareness and growth of pelvic pain treatments and introduces the principles of pelvic floor physical therapy."

In more detail, she began with stating that IBS can contribute to pelvic pain or even vice versa, and that proper physical therapy can greatly reduce IBS symptoms. This was something I had briefly heard before, but never considered it to be a big deal. Now I am completely rethinking eliminating a PT. Unfortunately, my bad experience with one of them left me feeling hopeless, but we will touch base on that in a moment.

Amy stated that women, who suffer from pelvic pain, should seek out a team of specialists, because there are more than likely several diagnoses that coincide with each other. Physicians, mental health providers, nutritionists, fitness trainers, physical therapists, and pelvic floor specialists are all important individuals to be considered for your "team." However, Amy stated that not all PTs are educated to treat pelvic pain, and as I mentioned above, I experienced this along my own journey, hindering me from seeking out another.

I had one good PT, who had the knowledge and skill set to work with my vaginismus and improve my symptoms, but the most recent PT had no clue what she was doing. She basically guessed her way through everything in my opinion and made things worse. Amy mentioned that this is extremely common. Many women go to a PT and have a similar negative experience. They then become discouraged because they are not getting results and stop going. However, it's not your body's fault for not getting those desired results, and it's important to stay hopeful and continue to find a PT that works with the pelvic floor.

Amy discussed that physical activity is extremely important for women who struggle with pelvic pain because it helps to get the blood circulating. Walking, yoga, elliptical machines, and Pilates are all great examples of physical activity. You need to make sure you are circulating the blood but not causing yourself pain. That's where part of the "team" comes into play. They can tell you what the best fitness plan for you is, since everyone's pain level and circumstances are different.

However, another thing that I learned from the interview is that biking is not a good form of physical activity for those who suffer from pelvic pain. This was new to me. I love to bike and even did a spinning/cycling class in college. However, biking can cause the PC muscles to tighten too much, making the pain and symptoms much worse.

Common myth: One myth that Amy introduced, and that I had also been told by my first PT, is that Kegel exercises are NOT GOOD for patients who suffer from vaginismus. The whole point of overcoming vaginismus is to learn to loosen the muscles, so it would not make much sense to tighten them even more. In fact, Kegel exercises can make things worse for these particular patients. However, if you are suffering from loose muscles, like after giving birth, then Kegel exercises are extremely important.

Chapter 10: Let's Talk About Boys

Vaginismus is not something I would wish on my worst enemy. It is unforgiving and drapes the individual who has it with depression and worry. Will it ever go away? Will my partner leave me? Why are they with me if I can't please them? Is all of it really my fault?

Believe it or not I have been asked all of these questions in one-way shape or form by guys that I have dated in the past. They made me feel like vaginismus was my fault, like everything was my fault, and I am still recovering to remove that trauma I felt from years of emotional abuse. I was so manipulated that I worked extra hard to please them because they threatened to leave me.

Boys have told me to get over it, to drink and make it go away, to lie back and pretend it feels good because it'll all be over soon, to not ruin their day because of it, even though on that day I was having a hard time listening to others talk about sex. I have been told that I simply lie there, that it's annoying or that since I can't have sex with them I should just pleasure them instead. I have been told it's annoying when I cry about it and to toughen up. Did they even realize that I would roll over every night and cry silently to myself, so that I didn't bother them?

I have asked boyfriends to stop talking about our sex life, like it's some amazing thing when it isn't, and all I got back was that I was being too dramatic. They never stopped…

I have been told I don't try hard enough. I was told by a boyfriend that he and a cousin were going to go to a strip club because he can't get any at home. I have even been told, while in the midst of tears, that the worst part about it is that I can't have make up sex after arguments, yet that didn't stop him from having sex with me anyways. All the while I cried, and, in that moment, I shut off all emotion.

After that night, I'm still trying to bring back that happy girl who loved romance. I miss the girl who loved to be loved. It's slowly coming back thanks to my amazing fiancé, but there is still much work to be done.

I understand that it's hard for guys to deal with vaginismus when their partner has it. I have read numerous books on how to talk to your partner when you have it, to understand what they are feeling inside, and to build a friendship with them to strengthen the bond. However, all my efforts were in vain. When your mom told you there is a difference between a boy and a man, she was right.

The individual/s above were all boys; too insensitive to understand that I was doing everything in my power to make them happy. Fighting back tears during sex so that they could enjoy themselves, while all the while I was screaming in pain on the inside and biting my tongue.

A man is someone who will be there for you during the hard times. Instead of watching you cry as he tells you everything that is wrong with you, not even once offering to give you a hug, a man will give you a shoulder to cry on and tell you that it's not your fault. A man will understand that you are doing everything you can to remove this evil enemy from you and he will be patient and respectful with you throughout that journey.

Chapter 11: The good, the bad and the ugly

By now, you've probably gained a pretty good grasp of vaginismus and how it can impact the daily lives of individuals who have it. Some days, I am happy with the help of the meds, but by the end of the day, I've used up all my energy and can't help but collapse with anxiety or depression. Other days, I struggle all day long to keep my composure at work and in public, so that I don't let on that I'm terribly depressed inside.

I still remember the first day I found out I had vaginismus. My mom took me to my gynecologist appointment, where they were going to give me the dilators. I kept silent the entire time, listening to every word the doctor was telling me, yet all the while I was shaking. It wasn't until my mom and I got back into the car that I opened the box of dilators and wept. My mom didn't know what to do at first. Give me space or give me a hug? Either way, I was overwhelmed because I was diagnosed with something that isn't easy to treat, during a time in my life where I was supposed to have fun and be care free.

Fast forward a few weeks later during my freshman year of college. A few girls that I went to high school with, who claimed to be my friends, started a rumor that I was sleeping around. Now, you can understand how emotionally traumatizing that was for me at that time. Just a few weeks before, I was diagnosed with this condition and now I am indiscreetly being told by old friends that I am a whore and being blocked on Facebook because they refused to tell me who said these nasty things. I felt so isolated, abused and embarrassed.

I wanted to share this story with you because it's not only boys that can be hurtful, but girls as well. I was always bullied in school, from first grade through my senior year of high school, and that grief can leave a mark. All those years of bullying gave me severe anxiety and depression, but it also taught me to be kind to others, especially because you have no idea what that person may be going through in their personal life.

Chapter 12: What it's like to have Vaginismus?
(real women, real stories)

It's not fun, I can tell you that. It's like a dark cloud hovering above you. The media and the lives we live today are also constantly reminding us how important sex is, through movies, music, books and magazines. For a long time, I resented vaginismus for taking away a part of me that I deserve to have. It's something that every normal person can do, yet I'm left behind in the shadows.

Every time I watch a romantic movie, I do become sad and tear up, yet can't stop watching it because it fills a void inside of me. I get sad when girlfriends talk about sex and their love life because I envy them and wish I could enjoy the same thing with my fiancé. I'm so happy for them and wish I could enjoy the "girl talk" like a normal friend, but afterwards, I go home and cry because I realize I'm losing some of the best years of my life with my own man.

I often feel abnormal, even though no one around me knows I have this problem. I worry that it will never go away and that I'll be stuck with this "curse" that past boys have told me I have. I have even recently turned to eating more because it's the only way I can get dopamine.

I also remember one day, years ago, when my mom had taped a recording of the Doctor Oz show because they were going to be talking about vaginismus. My mom had not seen it yet and was excited to watch it with me. However, when the doctor brought up the condition, everyone in the audience laughed, even the doctor. He said, "Yes, I know it sounds ridiculous and made up." I was heartbroken and disgusted. I turned it off immediately. Basically, he confirmed that I was abnormal in the public's eyes.

Even with a wonderful man by my side, there are many days where I curl up in bed and cry, unable to go outside for a whole day. Yet, I keep having to remind myself that I am not the vaginismus or the depression. I am a much stronger person than that and I need to remain positive that I will overcome this condition.

Listed below are other women who have graciously shared their stories with all of you. Through the pain, the triumphs, the struggles, these women have found courage to share their stories with the world. I hope this gives those of you who are reading this the strength to never give up hope and the understanding that you are not alone.

Stories from women who struggle with pelvic pain

R's Story

"I have had this [vaginismus] for nearly 5 years it has been a great bane in my life - but I'm in a much happier place, mentally. I hope to overcome it one day…not many people like to talk about it."

What advice would you give to women who are struggling with a similar condition? "To not blame themselves, to seek help as soon as they think something is not quite right, to be kind to themselves and remember it's a process and to try and to build a support system for those rough and down days." ~ R.

Jamie's Story

"One thing I have learned through the years is that having sex with my husband is painful at times. I really thought that this was always "just in my head" until I started reading my cousin's blog. For me, having sex at times is like my vagina is on fire. With every movement it feels like my inside is raw and that the walls are sandpaper. I would often cry and tell my husband to stop. He would get upset because he would think I did not want to spend time with him. This could be furthest from the truth. It is just painful and uncomfortable that it makes me not really want to have sex. I am content without it a lot because of the pain it causes me to have. There are a few lubricants out there that do help. I also have got to the point that I will share how I'm feeling with my husband, that way, we can work on a plan together. This to me, was normal until I started reading my cousins blog. I was finding myself relating to some of her experiences and it got me thinking and doing some research of my own. I am glad I did because now I realize that this does not define who I am. Yes, it is a big part that plays a part in my daily life but it's not the most important part. I want others to know they are not alone and to speak up. I have found my voice finally with all of this and I am glad I have. My advice would be to always trust yourself. If you think there is something wrong than trust it and go see someone before it gets too far out of control." ~ *Jamie*

M's Story

"Hey girl! I wanted to reach out and say you're so brave for sharing your story. A few weeks ago, I was struggling because I have endometriosis and having sex can get really painful. Emotionally, it's a rollercoaster and I feel like I can't do one of the most natural things in life. I was feeling alone and non of my friends or family have similar problems. That was the day you first shared your story, and I was so very grateful because I knew I was not alone. Thank you for your bravery and honesty! Last time I had sex I was in pain for two days…it just made it feel "real." Maybe you can relate to that moment?" ~ *M.*

Karlie's Story

"I just wanted to let you know how happy I was to come across your blog. Knowing that you aren't the only one in the world with this condition helps. I have been dealing with chronic hip pain, vaginismus, and pelvic floor dysfunction, along with depression and anxiety because of these issues, for the last five years. I would be happy to connect with you and exchange how we've dealt with everything. Looking forward to talking with you! When I went to the gynecologist for the first time, they were unable to perform the exam. I found out that I had an imperforate hymen. I then had this band of tissue surgically removed. The procedure is called a hymenotomy. After the surgery, when I tried insertion of any kind, is when the unbearable pain began. I went back into the doctor who performed the surgery and she diagnosed me with vaginismus caused from the trauma to the area from the previous surgery. This was in 2012 and I have been dealing with it ever since. I have tired many different things and have actually found slight relief just about a month ago.

Advice: "The best piece of advice I could give to women struggling with this type of pain would simply be to never give up. There are always going to be different doctors to see, different pelvic floor physical therapists to try, different treatment options, etc. Once you feel like you've exhausted all of your options, there will always be something else. A big part of it is your mindset. You have to want to get better before you can actually get better. I know this isn't easy, I am still struggling, but it will get better.

Perseverance and a little faith will take you a very long way." ~
Karlie, 25

T's Story

"...unfortunately I have vaginismus. I thought about trying
to start with dating about a year ago before I found out that I had
vaginismus. I'm just writing this to you to ask, do you think it's
even a good idea to start dating? I mean how can it even turn into a
legit relationship when the person finds out about the condition that
I have? It really sucks, because I see others around me enjoying sex
and having normal healthy sex lives like normal 19-year olds, while
I'm trying to figure out if I have enough time to dilate while my
roommate is in her biology class lol. I'm so sorry you had to go
through so much bullshit with this condition. It really freaking
sucks! When I first found out about it I cried for like two days and it
was all I could think about. Even now I think about it almost 80% of
the time. It makes me feel like I'm missing out on a lot and plus I'm
in my youth and I don't want to look back when I'm older and
remember nothing but pain and failed dilator attempts lol.

Having vaginismus sometimes makes it hard for me to even
start talking to guys to be quite honest. I guess it's cause I don't
know how they'll react to it. It really sucks hearing friends talk
about relationships and sex and complain about their Love lives
when it seems like it's still easier for them even with their hard
times. It seems so trivial compared to what I'm going through. Like
at least they don't have to worry about feeling less than because you
can't do something that's supposed to come naturally. It feels like

every other girl is automatically better because they can put things up their vagina with ease. I know that sounds ridiculous and I'm in no way less than, but it's hard to knock the feeling ya know. Hopefully I'll be able to update you on the progress and such because I really need a friend right now. My parents are great and are really supportive, but I feel like they think I make everything about sex and my vagina, but it sometimes really hard not to think about it because it's literally everywhere. Sex is everywhere, and I can't get over it because it seems like everyone is enjoying their bodies and I'm trapped in mine because it won't let me be.

Going to the gyno was an interesting experience to say the least. When they finally called me in, I had maybe like a 20 min talk with my gyno. I told her about my concerns with inserting tampons and she said she would try and see what's going on by examining me. This was when I started to panic on the inside. Luckily, she used only her fingers and a Q-tip. But let me tell ya, that Q-tip was a tragic experience, that's when I knew something was up. I was yelping on the table and she just wouldn't stop. I told her it hurt but she still kept going.

After that horrible experience, she finally told me I had vaginismus. She kind of glossed over it like it wasn't that big of a deal and didn't really give me any extra info on it. She was just like "oh yeah you have vaginismus, but you'll be fine". I was like "what the hell is a vaginismus?" But before I could even get the sentence out, she left. Poof, she was gone like a ghost. I sat there for like 2 mins wondering "what the fuck just happened?".

When I got out, I told my mom about it and she looked at me the same way I was looking when the gyno told me. When we got home, we both looked it up to see what it was. This was when it hit me how bad this condition could be. I was literally shooketh. I was shaking, and I started balling my eyes out. My mom told me that everything would be fine and she told me that she'd send me to another gyno since the one I went to was trash. I read article after article, I looked at videos with women who dealt with the conditions. I even made the horrible decision of reading the horrendous comments on YouTube of those videos.

The next gyno I went to was even worse. It's obvious that she didn't even know what vaginismus was. She basically told me to "just relax and to not even try to use tampons and let life happen." What the hell is that? It's like she was telling me it'll work itself out. She did mention that my hymen was covering the majority of my vaginal opening and that it's smaller than normal. That's the only useful info she gave me.

She [my mom] mentioned to me that maybe I could get help with seeing a physical therapist for my condition. When she mentioned that I thought "omg duh! How did I not think of that?" I mean I'm going to school for pelvic floor physical therapy. I don't know why that never crossed my mind. I guess you never think about getting physical therapy for your vagina. But when my mom mentioned that, it felt like I had a small glimpse of hope.

When I went to my first visit, I was a little nervous and on edge. I noticed that I was the only young-looking person in there and instantly felt like a failure. I felt the eyes looking at me like "what is this young girl doing in here?" Lol. When they finally called me in, I was nervous as hell. My palms were sweating, my legs are shaking and of course my vagina was clenching up. I went in and my therapist asked me the usual questions like: are you sexual active, have you experienced any sexual abuse, do you have any issues with masturbation or on a scale of one to ten, how bad is the pain. She made me take off my pants to examine me. To be honest, she was only able to do external. To this day, she still hasn't been able to do internal. I've only gone three times, but still.

I'm still struggling to be honest, but I'm actually considering a hymenotomy. I've looked down at my vagina with a mirror a few times and my whole is very tiny and I do feel that if I get the procedure it will help me get to where I want to be. It won't solve my issue completely, but I feel it'll get me started in the right direction once it done. My parents are 100% supportive and I'm thankful that they are willing to help me out no matter what, I've shared some pretty embarrassing information with them my whole life, they literally know everything about me, I've never hid anything from them. My mom is helping out with making this procedure happen and I'm looking forward to it. I'm still doing the exercises my PT has assigned me to do. Dilators are still killer, and I almost got caught with using them the other day lol. My roommate came in out of nowhere, with two of her friends. It's also gotten a bit harder to do that there as she always has this one friend who is constantly in our room with her. Thankfully I don't live far from my college so I just go home on the weekends and on night when I work so I get more alone time.

I hate this condition with a passion, but for some reason I think it's just what I needed. It's made me even more committed to going to college and becoming a pelvic floor specialist and even made me more comfortable with taking my clothes off down below and letting all out. I won't be a prisoner of vaginismus forever and neither will you. Maybe this was something I needed to gain even more experience to help others. I'm struggling but I'm also learning. One thing that I read that Fran Drescher from "the nanny" (I know weird right?) said was that, "sometimes the greatest gifts come in the ugliest packages." I have vaginismus and it sucks, and I'm gonna go through some rough days because of it but I two choices. To sit let it defeat me or to get off my ass and conquer and even learn from it while doing it. It's really hard trying to be positive and keep a good outlook on it. But it's taught me a few things about life. Life is not fair and there are things that you may come as easy to you as others. One way I've learned to kind of cope with it is by trying to look at greater picture and not the situation. You gotta have faith, because if you don't, you'll suffer..badly. I've been knocked down a lot by this condition in less than a year lol. I can't escape, and I feel trapped. But I feel like once I conquer it, I'll come out stronger than ever. And quite frankly, I feel like I'll be able to take anything that's thrown my way after that.

I'm gonna get through this and so are you.

Everyone has issues and this one is yours. No matter how many times that dilator just doesn't want to go in, or how many times you end the night of trying to have sex with your boyfriend in the bathroom crying with shower running, it's all going to be worth it in the end. I feel like vaginismus and similar conditions can be like gifts given in an ugly package. You become stronger, it can help you ween out assholes and scumbags, and most importantly it makes you more bold. I'm stilling dealing with vaginismus but I feel myself becoming more and more bold with the way I do things. I'm not afraid to tell people I'm in pain, I'm not afraid to advocate for myself and I'm not afraid to speak up. That's what I think is the most important thing. You can't let it bring you down and you have to be able to look at things in a more positive light. You get more creative in how you go around obstacles to succeed and see more results.

... even if times get rough and it seems like hope is gone, you have to keep trying, because that's what you would do with anything else in life. If it's something you want to overcome, doing something is better than doing nothing at all and giving up on when things don't go well. You have been willing to make a fool of yourself in order to be great, you have to be willing to come across people who will think you're crazy and tell them to that wrong to their face. You have to be willing to go through the worst before it even gets better. There's no easy way out, but what's you get out to the other side it'll be worth it, and it'll be so much to you because you had to go through so much to get there."

Advice: "Well, obviously I would start off by saying that they're not alone and it's not something that is going to be a forever struggle. There are solutions and there are ways to fix this issue. But I would emphasize that it's important to be brave enough to do what you can to fix your problem. It's going to be really tough and there's going to be times where you're say "I should give up and become a nun." But deep you'll know that's not really what you want. Comparing yourself to other women who don't have this issue also isn't going to help and it does nothing but make you feel worse." ~ *T., 19*

L. Jones' Story

"…in March 2017, I had an open myomectomy for uterine fibroids. Eight months later all heck broke loose. I started having sharp stabbing pain in my pelvic area left side. I thought it was ovaries. I endured the pain, as well as other symptoms from the fibroids that grew back. I felt horrible and in April 2018, I had a robotic myo to remove the new fibroids. I hoped the left side pelvic pain would decrease when adhesions were removed but nope. Here I am, 2 months post op and I have constant pain at the incision site from the first surgery. The doctor believes it's muscle issues. I started acupuncture and acupressure, which seems to help but not sure what else to do. I would suggest joining a support group like this one. If I had known about support groups prior to my first surgery, I would not be in the situation I am in. Knowledge is power and the best teachers are those who have experience. I would also encourage women to be encouraged and their number 1 advocate. Speak up, read and ask questions. Oh, and do not be afraid of getting 2nd, 3rd or 4th opinions." ~ *L. Jones, 42*

1. **What were you diagnosed with and at what age?** I was officially diagnosed at 33 with Endometriosis and then at age 37 I was diagnosed with Pelvic Floor Dysfunction.

2. **Were you self-diagnosed?** I always knew that something was right and that my symptoms were more than just period cramps.

3. **What did the doctors tell you about your condition?** I have seen several doctors over the course of many years. My symptoms were actually present at my first period which was age 9. Most of the doctors I saw had told me that it was just painful period cramps, that it was normal, and they would prescribe birth control bills or NSAIDS. The first surgery that I had to officially give me my diagnosis I was told by my surgeon that she had removed all of my lesions and that I shouldn't have further issues (unfortunately my symptoms returned 6 months later, and I had a second surgery 2 years later.

4. **Did they seem positive or come across negatively?** I feel that most of the doctors I spoke with in the beginning were not very educated on the disease, its symptoms or treatment. I continued to educate myself and search for doctors that were specialist and skilled in these areas. Through many doctors and years, I have finally found a team of doctors that understand the diagnose and have a positive overlook on the treatment plan.

5. **Did they teach you to use the dilators or simply hand them to you?** I am presently in treatment with Pelvic Floor Physical Therapy, were I am learning different techniques.

6. **What solution did doctors give you regarding your condition?** Most of the doctor I had saw in the past prescribed birth control pills, NSAIDS, made suggestions that pregnancy may help with the symptoms, some even suggested that it was in my head.

7. **How did the doctors make you feel emotionally?** Most of the time, I was so frustrated and exhausted with having to explain the same symptoms over and over and having them not be able to provide me with answers or make me feel as though my symptoms were no important. It wasn't until I found a team of doctors that I started to feel hopeful.

8. **What treatments have you tried?** 2 Surgeries, Pelvic Floor PT, Trigger Point Injections to the Pelvic Floor, Hip Steroid Injections, suppositories, creams, birth control pills, pain patches, pain medication, TENS units, CBD oil

9. **What advice would you give to other women struggling with this condition?** Never give up!!! This is not in your head, this is a whole-body condition, so all areas need to be balanced and healed. It takes a team, but you should always be the one in charge of your health. Listen to your body and learn what helps and what doesn't and always remember you are not alone! ~ *S. Gorny*

Elise's Story

"I was diagnosed at age 21 with primary vaginismus by an OB/GYN (1.5 years ago). However, my boyfriend and I had been googling pain with sex because we kept having unsuccessful attempts and were pretty sure that was what was going on. My OB/GYN told me what the condition was, said that it could be fully treated, and gave me a pamphlet with information. Because I was in college and my OB/GYN was at home, she didn't recommend any other resources.

At first, I thought it was going to be a straightforward process -- buy the dilators, do them, be cured. But I couldn't get the first dilator in. I tried and tried for months and got so discouraged. Finally, I decided to see a physical therapist (my first out of three). It was not a good experience. She was extremely condescending and physical therapy essentially consisted of weird leg and bowel massages by her, and me trying to insert a Q tip while she stepped out of the room. Obviously, I was there because I couldn't insert anything so...

I found a different physical therapist. I went to her for a few months, and she was much better. However, I still could not insert any of the dilators on my own. She focused a lot on the deeper muscles and I am pretty sure now that the issue is the entrance muscles.

I then moved across the country for graduate school and finally found a great physical therapist. She is very patient, and always has good suggestions about how to make at-home exercises better. I'm now on the third dilator after 6 months with her. Also, importantly, I found a psychological therapist who specializes in pelvic pain. Those two people combined have both been key for me.

Overall, doctors have been very friendly and generally positive about the condition, though I haven't been to an OB/GYN since I was diagnosed. It was my first pap smear at 17 that contributed significantly to my vaginismus so I'm waiting to do that again until I am more cured.

I wasn't deterred from getting into a relationship because I was already in one, and that is how I knew something was wrong. No males other than my boyfriend or dad (because he is helping pay for my various therapies) knows, so I can't really contribute to how guys have reacted. My boyfriend is nothing but loving and supportive, though it has taken him time to really understand what I am going through.

Here is some advice I would give to other women:

1) You CAN overcome this, no matter how hopeless you feel.

2) Seek physical therapy and psychological therapy, especially if you are having issues with avoidance, hopelessness feeling, lack of progress, etc. I waited way too long, thinking that I could power through. I couldn't.

3) No one really talks about how long or expensive of a journey this can be. I don't know what I thought -- most of the posts I read were people doing the dilators on their own, on a scale of weeks, but I am moving at a pace of months. My therapy is incredibly expensive, but it is worth the expense.

4) Find a female friend or two you can share your experiences with. Society as a whole needs to be more open about pelvic pain, and it will help you to not keep it bottled up.

5) Your motivation has to come from you, not from your partner. The more pressure you feel, the harder treatment it will be. This might require a lot of soul searching for you and your partner and very open communication, so no one develops resentment." ~ *Elise*

Taylor's Story

1. **What were you diagnosed with and at what age?**

I was diagnosed with vaginismus by my gynecologist around the age of 19.

2. **Were you self-diagnosed?**

I was not, as I previously mentioned my gynecologist is the one who diagnosed me. However, I could tell that something wasn't normal which is what made me see my doctor in the first place about the issue.

3. **What did the doctors tell you about your condition? Did they seem positive or come across negatively?**

I first went to my primary care physician who treated me for a yeast infection (that I did not have) and when I told her I was still having pain she referred me to a gynecologist. My gynecologist very quickly diagnosed me and set me up with a physical therapist. All of the doctors I saw were incredibly kind and supportive, I was also very young and clearly anxious so that may have also played a role. However, I do have a vivid memory of the woman at the checkout counter of my doctor's office stating (loudly for everyone to hear, including other patients) that she thought it was "weird" I had been referred to a physical therapist by a gynecologist as she had never seen that before. (I was so mortified that I ended up crying in my car. If I had been the head strong woman I am now I would have torn that lady a new one.)

4. **Did they teach you to use the dilators or simply hand them to you?**

My physical therapist recommended a dilator kit to me and provided some information on how to use them although it wasn't as in depth as I would have really liked. I honestly didn't use them as much as I probably should have and mostly because I didn't know what I was doing. However, I could have (and probably should have) spoken up about that to my PT and she would have been more than happy to work with me to make it work.

5. **What solution did doctors give you regarding your condition?**

The only real solution a doctor gave me was physical therapy which did help in some aspect but eventually the problem kept reoccurring. I went to physical therapy at a few different points in my life but could never maintain a pain-free sex life. I am a survivor of childhood sexual abuse which I thought I had moved on from, but it wasn't until I start counseling for sexual dysfunction that I really started to overcome the vaginismus.

6. **How did the doctors make you feel emotionally?**

I never had a bad experience with any of my doctors regarding the condition. I typically only see women doctors, and all have been sympathetic and supportive.

7. **What treatments have you tried?**

I have tried physical therapy, psychotherapy, muscle relaxers, and medical marijuana.

8. **Were you deterred from getting into a relationship because of your condition?**

I have been in a committed long-term relationship for roughly 7 years, so I was already with my partner when this problem started occurring. He has been nothing but supportive of me and understanding throughout our entire relationship.

9. **What were some things guys have said to you about your condition?**

My partner has always been kind and supportive. However other guys that I have mentioned this to usually respond with "that doesn't sound like a problem to me" which is horribly invalidating and frustrating. Sex is supposed to be about both partners enjoyment and pleasure.

10. **What advice would you give other women struggling with this condition?**

I would tell women that it is a process and a journey, and it can take a lot of hard work to overcome it. I was frustrated a lot and had to learn how to talk about myself and my vagina in a positive way instead of letting my negative emotions get the best of me. It's hard work but it doesn't have to be a forever problem. ~ *Taylor*

1. **What were you diagnosed with and at what age?**

    Officially diagnosed at age 22

2. **Were you self-diagnosed?**

    Initially I self-diagnosed around age 20-21, but I was still in denial so I didn't really claim it.

3. **What did the doctors tell you about your condition?**

    The first few doctors told me that it was all in my head and it must be trauma-related (which it wasn't) and then another doctor told me it was because I carry all my stress in my vagina? Another told me it was all the years of being brought up around the church that condemned sex and it was too engrained in my mind that it was wrong.

4. **Did they seem positive or come across negatively?**

    I would say it was split.

5. **Did they teach you to use the dilators or simply hand them to you?**

    Only the last one told me kind of how it worked, but not real direction

6. **What solution did doctors give you regarding your condition?**

    They told me to "relax". Another told me about dilators and gave anti-anxiety meds (that i've only taken once) and some numbing cream (never used that either)

7. **How did the doctors make you feel emotionally?**

    Felt pretty apathetic and like I was insane sometimes

8. **What treatments have you tried?**

"Relaxing" getting drunk. dilators

9. **Were you deterred from getting into a relationship because of your condition?**

oh yeah. multiple times.

10. **What were some things guys said to you about your condition?**

That sex was an important part of the relationship and that it was all in my head and not real and I had so much going for me but it was too much to handle. another that they would stick around if I worked on it, but it seemed like I didn't want to get better. that I was playing the victim and I had all the control over it

11. **What advice would you give to other women struggling with this condition?**

I would say that you need to start with small goals and make sure getting better is what is really important. you don't have to get it done fast or right away. That it's hard and you will want to give up, but one day it will be easy. It'll be like training for a marathon and the finish line is worth it. And DO NOT have any shame about it. It's not anyone else's business, but don't be afraid to talk about it. *~Krista*

For a select few of these women, the doctors they initially sought out were uneducated or unhelpful about the condition. Most agreed that female sexual dysfunction is often not discussed, and that something needs to change to acknowledge these issues more regularly. Many of the women were already in relationships where their partners were patient; however, a few were even afraid to enter a relationship in fear that boys would not be understanding of their condition. All of these women gave similar advice for others struggling with pelvic pain. Their advice was to be patient with yourself and stay positive. Find a support group to talk with and know that you can overcome this condition with hard work. Don't ever give up on yourself!

Story from a man who struggles from pelvic pain

Sometimes, it is not just women who struggle with pelvic pain, but men as well. Here is one story from a male who was gracious enough to let me interview him on his condition.

Anonymous' Story

"As a man with erectile dysfunction I've never felt any pelvic pain. The best way to explain it is like a numbness in the crotch region. Mainly due to a lack of blood flow when I am turned on but cannot get an erection.

It has an impact every second of every day. When you see the beautiful woman, you want to ask on a date the ED is always in the back of your mind. Even more on a date when you know the woman your taking out wants sex. When it comes down to getting intimate you know it's probably not going to happen.

I am not sure what or how this was caused. I remember as a young teen the pressure that was felt to lose your virginity between your peers. I was never good with the ladies, so it did take me quite a while to and it's very possible that there is some subconscious anxiety tied to anything sexual I do. Our culture is so obsessed with sex all while condemning it at the same time. I believe some anxiety for sexual dysfunction in myself and in most men stems from a cultural expectation to be the alpha male and to lead and dominate in the bedroom. Men are expected to take that role. When a cultural expectation like that is set it can bring up performance anxiety consciously or subconsciously. This is an issue that plagues many more men in our society than we know but what man is willing to swallow his pride to admit this?

I have told and not told some women if I believe I am only engaging in a one-night stand. If I can't get an erection I usually blame it on consuming to much alcohol. Sometimes I will go to the doctors and get erection meds and if I know I'm going to get intimate for a night I will sneak away and take one and this normally work. Any long-term relationship I have had I have always told my partner and while they say they understand sometimes they feel it is there fault for not being able to turn me on. Sometimes my condition makes my significant other feel ugly or unloved which is never the case.

I have gone through many bouts of depression over this. The inability to get sexual when I need to creates an anxious depression for me. I feel like I have missed out on so much. I began taking anxiety medication almost a year ago and this has helped me quite a bit. Unfortunately, a side effect to the meds makes my ED worse. I have been working so much I haven't had time to meet women. I do one-night stands on occasion but I'm really not a fan of them. My ED makes it very hard to get turned on unless I am very comfortable and have feelings for the woman I am getting intimate with. in my early 20s I felt the most anger and depression over this. Looking back the anger and depression stole a few great years of my life. the moments I look back on where I was unhappy in the moment now I memorize as some of my life's great moments. I may have not been able to have sex at the time but the places I've traveled and seen and the great people I have had the privilege of meeting and the crazy situations I put myself in will forever make me smile. Knowing this now has helped me relax and better enjoy the moment now. My ED may always haunt me, but I have learned I am in control. I don't have to let the anger resentment and depression take over. All I can do is live my life to the best of my ability and go after what I want out of my life.

The ED makes me cautious about getting into a relationship. It's very difficult to navigate and most women have trouble handling it I think. I honestly don't put forth the energy and effort to be in a relationship because it is a scary thing to do. In today's society, we switch partners so fast sometimes and it is very hard to deal with emotionally. I may not show it but rejection really bothers me." ~*Anonymous*

When asked how Anonymous thinks ED is similar to women with vaginismus he said, "I wish I had a solid answer. As a man, I can't really understand the pain you are going through during sex. I believe the mental damage it does to a man and a woman are almost exactly the same however. I felt alone for a very long time and sometimes I still do. Finding people like you and others to talk to about it has helped me quite a bit. I think having a small portion of your book dedicated to males with sexual dysfunction would be a good thing to make it known both genders suffer. I've often wondered if dating a woman with vaginismus would be a good thing for myself and her since we would both have in common the sexual dysfunction."

His enlightening and courageous story opens up a whole new topic regarding pelvic pain in men. They experience it the same way we do and even have an added layer of anxiety because of society's expectation for them to take charge in the bedroom. Even though he does not have similar physical symptoms as women, he is still experiencing the same mental and emotional struggles that all of us face when dealing with pelvic pain. For those men reading this book, who also struggle with ED, I hope this finds you and provides you with comfort. Know that you are not alone in this either.

Stories from men whose partners have pelvic pain

Every person has a story to tell and, while pelvic pain physically affects the women, it also emotionally affects the men in the relationship. However, not every man is the same in how he responds to his partner's pain. Not only is it informative to read the perspective of those who struggle with the condition, but let's read a few stories from partner's perspectives. Some have similarities and differences as you read along, but always keep in mind that a supportive partner is one who is willing to be patient with you to help you overcome your condition.

"Have lived with a partner with vaginismus (or some similar condition) for approx. 16 of the last 20 years. We met in grad school...have been married for 10 years. She has been my only partner.

She does not claim any past abuse. Neither of us come from religious households. She presents to the world as a sex-positive feminist (which makes me inwardly chuckle, just a bit).

She has refused to seek a diagnosis for twenty years, no interest in any form of therapy or counseling. When I have brought the issues up (maybe once a year), it's a teary emotional wall. I've brought up the term 'vaginismus', I assume she's done some internet reading on it herself but has never brought up the topic herself. Most days, it's all just ignored.

Feelings?

Dismissed and taken-for-granted come to mind. That something is an issue for me but (supposedly) not really an issue for her means it's not an issue worth examining. There are some fairly cutting jokes between us that a) I'd leave her if someone else came along and b) no one else would ever come along. I'd feel pretty damned flattered if she'd seek some change in the situation.

Isolated. Whether she wants to discuss or not, it's entirely her right to discuss her pain with female friends, counselors, doctors, whomever she would wish to (and I'd hope she would). For me, since it's not "my secret" to share (and male stoicism being what it is), I'd feel like I was outing someone else's secret to bring this up to any of my friends. As such, for twenty years I have not shared it with anyone save anonymously.

Curious. In that I've never had 'normal' sex, but it's so prevalent in the culture, yeah, I think about it a lot. You can talk about non-trad sex being just as good, and it may well be, or decide intellectually that you'd still love a partner with other physical/sexual inabilities... but it won't stop you from being curious about what all the fuss is about.

Also, tied up in the mix, at some point in our 30s, I got bit a little by the baby bug. I was doing well enough job-wise and friends started having families and thus I too was interested (she never was). I/we are too darned old for that now, but it's emotionally hard to deal with families and children, and I mostly avoid situations where I'd interact with kids as a result." ~ *Anonymous, 43*

D's Story

1. **What type of pelvic pain condition does your partner have?** Vaginismus and Vulvodynia are the ones I can remember, I think she's been given a few other diagnoses, but I forget the names of them, sorry! I can ask her if you need more clarification

2. **Does it affect your relationship? If so, how?** It does affect our relationship. It's hard to say exactly how as we've never had a relationship without it. It causes her a lot of anxiety and she used to worry that she wasn't enough for me (though I think that part has mostly gone away). It definitely affects our sex life, as we're constantly navigating what is okay at any given moment.

3 & 4. **Are you bothered by it in any way?** It is absolutely frustrating. I hate that my girlfriend has to deal with being in pain all the time, and that we can't always do things we both want to do because of it. I hate how it makes her feel inadequate and anxious and frustrated and guilty and not normal.

5. **Do you talk about the condition with her?** Absolutely. Communication is very important. We talk about it all the time.

6. **Have you ever sought out information on your own? If so, what was it and why?** Yes! I have read about the condition for my knowledge, I've read a few blogs. I looked for support groups in our area. I also subscribe to the vaginismus and vulvodynia subreddits. I think it really helps me understand what she is dealing with to read the stories of other people in the same situations.

7. **Do you help her with the dilators? Do you go to her with PT?** I have before but generally she wanted to do it on her own. She has stopped dilating since we have been able to have penetrative sex. I want her to continue with in but she's been in a bit of a rut for a while in terms of doing things to help herself. She made a lot of progress very quickly in the beginning and when things slowed down she lost the motivation to keep up with those things (dilating, stretching, etc.) I understand that this is not uncommon and try my best to be supportive.

She stopped going to PT because it was too expensive. I never went with her, but that was mostly due to the fact that we are both very busy and live about an hour apart.

8. **How do you help her with her condition?** I do my best to be supportive and listen to her. I encourage her to seek help and do things that I think will help her wellbeing. I have been with her for a few doctors' appointments if I can. I do my best to let her know she is loved and her condition does not affect that in any way.

9. **What do you think or say when guys become angry at their partner for having this condition?** It makes me angry that anyone would react that way. It is in no way their fault and what they have dealt with and have to continue dealing with is much worse than not being able to have sex whenever you want. I think this response comes from entitlement and anyone who gets angry at their partner for this should not continue to be a partner as they don't have anyone's interests in mind but their own.

10. **Does she often feel insecure or guilty with her condition? How do you help her then?** Absolutely! I try to tell her or show her that she has nothing to feel guilty or insecure about and that I'm there for her and it does not bother me at all.

11. **Are you both able to get intimate? This does not mean sex, but can be hand holding, cuddling, etc. If you can't, how does that make you feel?** We can! We hold hands and cuddle all the time! In terms of sexual intimacy, we adjust based on her pain levels at the moment. It can be difficult to navigate but we communicate well and do what we can. We can occasionally have penetrative sex, depending on how she's doing at any given moment, though this didn't happen until about 9 months or so into our relationship. She generally has a harder time getting in the mood but she says I'm good at helping her out with that :)

12. **Does she also struggle with anxiety or depression?**
Yes! Both! I don't think that it is completely due to her pelvic pain
issues but it definitely doesn't help.

13. **What type of help is she receiving?** Currently she is
not receiving much help. In the beginning of her journey to heal she
had a huge amount of help from Dr. Echenberg from the institute for
pelvic and sexual pain
(http://www.instituteforwomeninpain.com/about-dr.-echenberg) he
was an amazing help and did so much for her. They are still in
contact and she is on a slew of drugs he prescribed. She used to go
to PT but that stopped due to finances. She was regularly seeing a
therapist and she still sees her occasionally but it's pretty infrequent
these days. She also writes a blog about it occasionally and I think
that is very cathartic for her.

14. **Are you seeking help of any kind for yourself?
(therapy, forums, etc.?)** I read the subreddits I mentioned earlier,
but other than that. Not really.

15. **When did she tell you she had this condition?** It was
before we really got serious. We had made out a couple times, but
she was always hesitant to do more (shocker), so I think it was
maybe our 3rd real date (we were friends for a while before dating).
She has a much better memory for the timing of things. If you'd like
to talk to her I'd be happy to give you her info. I'm sure she'd be
happy to talk.

16. How did you respond? I think I was kind of confused. I
asked a lot of questions. But, mostly I think I just kinda said ok, and
that I still wanted to do what we were doing. ~ D.

R's Story

1. **What type of pelvic pain condition does your partner have?**

   I think they're called Vulvodynia and Vaginismus

2. **Does it affect your relationship? If so, how?**

   No not at all, it's not all about sex

3. **Would you say you are bothered by it in any way?**

   It bothers me that it hurts her, it's more of me being bothered because she's in pain.

4. **Does it make you depressed, angry or frustrated at times?**

   It's frustrating for me to see her to have this. It frustrates me because it distresses her.

5. **Do you talk about the condition with her?**

   Yeah we do, we talk about it frequently and I go to doctor and hospital appointments with her, but that's more for support.

6. **Have you ever sought out information on your own? If so, what was it and why?**

   No, we both look into things together, but I haven't looked into anything myself. We've looked into what the condition is and the symptoms, we've tried to rule out conditions, so we know what to tell the doctor

7. **Do you help her with the dilators? Do you go with her to PT?**

   I don't help her directly, she prefers to use her dilators alone. I feel it's an independent thing for her as she is in control of her pain. It seems too sensitive for me to be too involved with, wouldn't want to hurt her. I'd help her if she asked though

8. **How do you help her with her condition?**

I've learnt to be patient and take things at her pace, let her be in control.

9. **What do you think or say when guys become angry at their partner for having this condition?**

I've never met any other guy with a partner with vulvodynia, but I'd tell them you need to support her with the issue. It's not like she's doing it on purpose, it's through no fault of her own and she needs support.

10. **Does she often feel insecure or guilty with her condition? How do you help her then?**

Yeah in the past she's said she's felt guilty, but I told her not to worry about it. It's not her fault and she's trying her best to sort it.

11. **Are you both able to get intimate? This does not mean sex, but can be hand holding, cuddling, etc. If you can't, how does that make you feel?**

Yeah, we do other things instead of 'PIV' (Penis in Vagina).

12. **Does she also struggle with anxiety or depression?**

I know she gets anxious if we attempt PIV

13. **What type of help is she receiving?**

Not a lot! The NHS and doctors aren't helping the situation, they just want to put her on medication and aren't properly treating the problem. She's been to multiple doctors and had so many appointments and they just pass her around because nobody knows what to do with her condition. She's currently working through dilators but up until this month (we've been together 4 years) there hasn't been a lot of help from doctors.

14. **Are you seeking help of any kind for yourself? (therapy, forums, etc.?)**

No, nothing. I'm not aware of forums or help for partners with vulvodynia.

15. **When did she tell you she had this condition?**

She discovered she had it when we first tried to have sex, in the first year we were together.

16. **How did you respond?**

At first, I was frustrated but due to my age I had eventually realized it wasn't her fault that she had this condition. ~ R.

Anonymous' Story

1. **What type of pelvic pain condition does your partner have?**

She has a combination of vaginismus, endometriosis and one more issue that I sadly can never remember the name of. It all depends on which doctor we go to, as none of them can agree.

2. **Does it affect your relationship? If so, how?**

It very much affects our relationship, it not only causes our sex life to have long periods of nothing, it gives her massive anxiety whenever anything sexual is brought up, causing consistent strain. It goes in waves typically.

3. **Would you say you are bothered by it in any way?**

I am bothered, it is frustrating and depressing, but I know that it is even worse for her, and I have no plans on giving up.

4. **Does it make you depressed, angry or frustrated at times?**

It makes me depressed and frustrated, never angry, and never at her, more just in general.

5. **Do you talk about the condition with her?**

We discuss it fairly consistently, constantly seeking new information, potential new treatments and ways for us to work around it as a couple.

6. **Have you ever sought out information on your own? If so, what was it and why?**

Absolutely. I've searched my way around a lot, and a few of the suggestions I have found have helped a little.

7. **Do you help her with the dilators? Do you go with her to PT?**

Neither of these things have been offered to us, and we aren't in a situation where we can afford dilators ourselves, but I would gladly help with either.

8. **How do you help her with her condition?**

I always try to remain level headed, and I try my very best to never let her see if it's upsetting me. I have done all I can to reinforce that it is absolutely fine and that I am absolutely fine with it and that it will never make me love her less.

9. **What do you think or say when guys become angry at their partner for having this condition?**

I've never personally talked to someone in the same situation as us, so I couldn't say from experience. It does sound ridiculous to be angry at your partner for something out of their control though, and that is no way to have a relationship.

10. **Does she often feel insecure or guilty with her condition? How do you help her then?**

Fairly consistently. I always try to reinforce that it's not her fault, and that I am happy no matter what. Sometimes we browse the vaginismus or sex subreddits together because she finds it soothing.

11. **Are you both able to get intimate? This does not mean sex, but can be hand holding, cuddling, etc. If you can't, how does that make you feel?**

We are. We have had periods of little to no intimacy because we both felt very bad about the lack of sex, but after discussion we have done our best to make sure that doesn't happen again.

12. **Does she also struggle with anxiety or depression?**

She struggles with anxiety and depression, but not as disorders, more in the way most people become depressed or anxious.

13. **What type of help is she receiving?**

Very little currently. She has switched birth control method to see if that helps, other than that almost all help is done by each other, and consistently working on it.

14. **Are you seeking help of any kind for yourself? (therapy, forums, etc?)**

For myself? No.

15. **When did she tell you she had this condition?**

About 1 or 2 weeks after us officially calling it a relationship.

16. How did you respond?

I was incredibly hurt, because she revealed that every time we had sex until then very much hurt her, and that she only did it because she didn't want me to leave or think less of her. Hurting people isn't in my nature, and I felt terrible knowing that I had been hurting her almost daily for weeks. ~*Anonymous*

Kevin's Story

1. What type of pelvic pain condition does your partner have?

My partner has an involuntary tightening of her pelvic floor muscles which can lead to an intense burning sensation during penetration. There were times where it was physically painful for me as well as we would sometimes begin penetration and then she would involuntarily tighten around me.

2. Does it affect your relationship? If so, how?

It has definitely caused some frustration in our relationship but overall, I think we've only grown stronger as we worked through it together. It means that we have to be more mindful during our intimacy and that we have to keep in mind that sometimes penetration just isn't going to happen.

3. Would you say you are bothered by it in any way?

At first, I was bothered by it because we didn't understand why it was happening. We had a very satisfying sex life up until the onset of the vaginismus and it started deteriorating fairly rapidly.

4. **Does it make you depressed, angry or frustrated at times?**

I don't think it ever made me depressed or angry but there was definitely frustration. We went to different colleges about an hour apart and only had time to see each other once or twice a month. If during those times we weren't able to have penetrative sex it meant waiting another 2-3 weeks before we could even try again. It definitely dampened both of our spirits during unsuccessful attempts and led to decreased physical intimacy overall.

5. **Do you talk about the condition with her?**

We talk about her condition all the time! In the beginning neither of us knew what was happening so we would try to talk about it without the correct tools. Once she was diagnosed we were able to have very productive discussion over what it is and what's happening. We absolutely approached this problem as a team and I tried to be as supportive as I possibly could!

6. **Have you ever sought out information on your own? If so, what was it and why?**

Before we really knew what was happening I tried posting questions on /r/sex but unfortunately this was ~4 years ago and the topic wasn't discussed or known as much as it is today. Once we had an official diagnosis I looked at forums and articles to try to figure out how I could help her and how I could be more supportive.

7. **Do you help her with the dilators? Do you go with her to PT?**

Luckily there was a physical therapist who specialized in female pelvic floor issues at my university's hospital (University of Michigan if it matters). I went to every physical therapy appointment with her and was always in the room with her for support. Her physical therapist was an incredible source of information and she did a great job at making us both feel comfortable. Once we were tasked with dilator work I did help whenever I could. It was important for the exercise for her to do it on her own as well as for me to help at times. We went to physical therapy for about 8-10 months once a month before we felt like we started to get a handle on the vaginismus. Unfortunately, due to our busy college schedules, and the fact that we weren't able to see each other very often things started to regress. After a few unsuccessful months we went back to physical therapy to try to get back on track. We again fell into the same issues after another ~6 months of therapy but had to end due to our impending graduations and eventual move out of state. We did however, feel that we had the tools to continue on our own especially since we were going to be living together. After about a year of little success things started to get frustrating again (for both of us). She expressed many times how difficult it was because she "just wanted to have sex but her body wouldn't let her" it definitely took a toll on her emotions and self-confidence and was one of the reasons she started to go to therapy at her new grad school. We again, got extremely lucky and she started seeing a therapist who specialized in sexual dysfunction and made her feel comfortable enough to bring up this topic. Her therapist eventually suggested that I come in for a group session and I was very excited to start participating! I think the psychotherapy together really helped push us over the edge and helped us communicate better and more openly about this topic. It honestly didn't take many therapy sessions together before we started seeing huge improvements! Since the largest dilator didn't quite match up to our goal (not helping things)... in addition to dilator work we had "homework" that was to attempt a small amount of penetration with me laying still on my back and her lowering herself onto me from an upright position (only up to the vaginal entrance) and hold it, we did this about three times a week before moving on. After those successful attempts our next assignment was to try to go a little deeper. These practices were not supposed to be sexual and it was important that they were seen as "work" not "pleasure". Well, once we found that we were able to go deeper things moved pretty quickly and we were able to have penetrative sex after just one "homework" session. It seemed to us that the years of physical therapy had paid off and all we needed help with was getting over a mental block. We still take things slow and meet with our therapist semi-regularly, but things are definitely almost where we want them to be! In addition to the vaginismus the sex-therapy has completely transformed the way we communicate with each other during sex. We were definitely extremely good at communicating before and never really fight or argue (to the point that our friends say it sickens them) but if we saw this much good from seeing a therapist together I think it's something that everyone should do! She also helped us pinpoint what the likely cause of the vaginismus and why it started to show up when it did (there was nothing that we hadn't talked about before, but we were finally able to put the pieces together in a meaningful way).

8. **How do you help her with her condition?**

I try to be as patient as possible. I reassure her that I know it's not her fault and that while it can be frustrating I don't resent or in any way. I know that she wants the ordeal to be over with as much as I do and I did my best to let her know that we're in this together and that we will get through it! I also tried to go to every therapy appointment that I could and try everything that she suggested. We're a couple and this is a problem that we both need to learn how to work out.

9. **What do you think or say when guys become angry at their partner for having this condition?**

Other guys are definitely an interesting issue for me. I found it strange when I was praised by our physical therapist for being at every appointment or by our psychotherapist for being so supportive and willing... Why wouldn't someone want to support their partner? If a guy becomes angry over this issue I think they just truly don't understand the problem or there are other underlying issues. It's important to realize that you are a couple, you are both working on the same team and need to work with each other rather than against each other. It shouldn't ever become "me vs you", it should be "us vs the problem". I would tell guys who are angry to please please be patient with their partner, it's just as frustrating (if not more) for them as it is for you. Another thing I'd like to bring attention to is the general attitude towards this issue. We are both very open people and pretty much talked to anyone who was curious about this issue and our sex life. Many times I would explain the problem as "involuntary tightness" and guys would respond "doesn't sound like a problem to me hahahaha".... To which I would (usually) refrain from cracking a size joke at their expense and instead very seriously explain that sex (if possible) is physically painful for her and at times physically painful for me. I would ask them why they would ever want their partner to feel pain during sex (unless they and their partner are into that but that's a completely different topic, not a medical issue, and not the point). I never had a bad response from a guy after explaining in more detail what the issue is and how difficult it's been to deal with.

10. **Does she often feel insecure or guilty with her condition? How do you help her then?**

She has definitely told me that she feels inadequate, guilty, or incompetent. Much like my response in Q8 I reassure her that I know it's not her fault, we're both working at this together, and my number one priority is her being comfortable and happy. I tell her that I know how hard she's working and that I know how frustrating it is for her but that we're going to get through it and have lots of amazing and beautiful sex together once we're past it.

11. **Are you both able to get intimate? This does not mean sex, but can be hand holding, cuddling, etc. If you can't, how does that make you feel?**

We are able to be intimate. We have almost always been all over each other and are constantly holding hands and cuddling. During the most frustrating periods of dealing with vaginismus our intimacy definitely took a hit, but I think it's only because it reminded us of what we can't do. We found other ways to have fun and pleasure each other without penetration, that was probably the most important part of this. Just because we couldn't have penetrative sex like we used to didn't mean that we could take care of each other's physical needs in other ways. We also had to keep in mind that although we couldn't have penetrative sex, it was something we were actively working on and something that would happen eventually.

12. **Does she also struggle with anxiety or depression?**

She used to struggle a lot with depression and anxiety during her undergraduate years but has currently worked through her battle with depression. She is still working through her anxiety and takes medication to help cope. The depression/anxiety wasn't a cause or effect of the vaginismus but all of the issues working together had a way of making things more difficult to deal with.

13. **What type of help is she receiving?**

We were seeing a physical therapist and then after moving started to see a therapist who specializes in sexual dysfunction and has been treating her anxiety along with her vaginismus. Both methods of treatment were helpful in their own ways and I definitely think we were able to see such sudden progress in our fight against it due to both approaches. I think it's important to stress that we went about 4/5 years with seeing minimal improvements until we finally "broke the penetration barrier" and have been seeing rapid progression ever since.

14. **Are you seeking help of any kind for yourself? (therapy, forums, etc.?)**

As I mentioned before I went to every physical therapy appointment and joined her for couples and solo sessions with her sexual dysfunction therapist. In addition to this I did seek online forums to try to educate myself better about this condition. It was really important for us to stay together on this and both learn and share as much as possible. Communication is key!

15. **When did she tell you she had this condition?**

We first met in high school and were able to have sex without issue for about 2 years. Her vaginismus crept up on us in the form of burning during penetration and pain and discomfort during sex. Neither of us knew what was happening so we had to research the issue together. After much frustration and many dead-ends she was finally diagnosed with vaginismus and we were able to begin solving a problem that we had a name for.

16. **How did you respond?**

I had to be as supportive and understanding as possible. This was an issue that affected both of us, was frustrating for both of us, and one that we could get through together. *~Kevin*

Randy's Story

1. **What type of pelvic pain condition does your partner have?** She has vaginismus. Unable to get even her pinky finger into her vagina.

2. **Does it affect your relationship? If so, how?** We are no longer together, but when we were, it made us unable to

have penetrative sex. It also made her wildly jealous of all women I had slept with prior to her.

3. **Would you say you are bothered by it in any way?** I mean, I enjoy fucking, and missed it. But for the year I was with her, I was frankly able to stave off the challenge of being unable to fuck by dreaming of the day her therapy worked and I could fuck her. (that day never came)

4. **Does it make you depressed, angry or frustrated at times?** Yeah, it did. Particularly because I was polyamorous before we met, and her vaginismus-induced anxieties about other women made it impossible for us to be nonmonogamous. Thus, I was captive in a situation where I could not fuck. That drove me kind of crazy.

5. **Do you talk about the condition with her?** Often enough, but I tried not to take on a "therapy" role.

6. **Have you ever sought out information on your own? If so, what was it and why?** Yep, I followed /r/vaginismus and read a fair bit about the condition.

7. **Do you help her with the dilators? Do you go with her to PT?** She never used dilators while I knew her, though I purchased a couple for her. No PT because she did not have health insurance that was at all separate from her very overprotective, possibly abusive mother.

8. **How do you help her with her condition?** I guess I didn't. I told her she really needed to help herself.

9. **What do you think or say when guys become angry at their partner for having this condition?** I've never met one, but I'd have mixed feelings. On one hand, it's a dick move to be angry, but at the same time, it's really really challenging to be dating someone you can't have conventional sex with. Sometimes, that challenge drives you to anger.

10. **Does she often feel insecure or guilty with her condition? How do you help her then?** Yes she feels insecure about her condition. She says all other women I've ever slept with got a more "real" experience of me. Some of my poly lovers who I've talked about when drunk because I am an open person, she'll bring up during fights and cry and tell me to get back with one of them since she's "forever a virgin" etc. etc.

11. **Are you both able to get intimate? This does not mean sex, but can be hand holding, cuddling, etc. If you can't, how does that make you feel?** Yeah, we get intimate. I try to eat her out, but she takes longer and longer to cum because she is guilty that I can't fuck her. She'll go down on me but feels a sense of obligation about it that feels sort of nasty. Our sex life is not very good, mostly because of guilt and obligation... honestly, without those feelings, it could be great.

12. **Does she also struggle with anxiety or depression?** Yes, she is extremely depressed and anxious, and those conditions are intimately tied up with her vaginismus. She

cannot get out of bed often, she cannot work, she cannot do anything she likes doing. I am afraid she will kill herself sometimes.

13. **What type of help is she receiving?** None. Her mother will judge and follow her if she gets any type of therapy, and pressure her therapists to divulge information about her case to her. She is too poor and unemployable for any type of health insurance.

14. **Are you seeking help of any kind for yourself? (therapy, forums, etc.?)** No. Breaking up with her was my form of helping myself, sadly enough. The whole thing is horrible. I am also poor and uninsured.

15. **When did she tell you she had this condition?** When I tried to finger her the first night we met.

16. **How did you respond?** By not proceeding any further in fingering her and instead going down on her. *~Randy*

Anonymous' Story

1. **What type of pelvic pain condition does your partner have?** PIV is difficult. I have a small penis but can still only get about half in.

2. **Does it affect your relationship? If so, how?** Getting better. On the upside my (lack of) size isn't an issue as it has been with other women.

3. **Would you say you are bothered by it in any way?** Not going to lie, I would prefer to be able to go deeper.

4. **Does it make you depressed, angry or frustrated at times?** Dealing with it. Obviously, it's not her fault and we are making progress.

5. **Do you talk about the condition with her?** Yes lots

6. **Have you ever sought out information on your own? If so, what was it and why?** Yes, Google etc. and checked vaginismus group on Reddit, talked to a couple of women from there.

7. **Do you help her with the dilators?** Toys yes.

8. **How do you help her with her condition?** As above

9. **What do you think or say when guys become angry at their partner for having this condition?** That would be selfish

10. **Does she often feel insecure or guilty with her condition? How do you help her then?** At first but I think were past that now.

11. **Are you both able to get intimate? This does not mean sex, but can be hand holding, cuddling, etc. If you can't, how does that make you feel?** We can.

12. **Does she also struggle with anxiety or depression?** No

13. **what type of help is she receiving?** As above

14. **When did she tell you she had this condition?** First time we had sex.

15. **How did you respond?** I'd never heard of the condition before so listened/learnt. Bottom line is we've found lots of things beyond PIV which has definitely been a positive.

Also, I have no insecurity about my small penis - it clearly works better for us! ~*Anonymous*

Anonymous' Story

1. **What type of pelvic pain condition does your partner have?**

    Vaginismus

2. **Does it affect your relationship? If so, how?**

    Yes, it greatly affects our relationship. We have been together for four and a half years, got married last month, and have been unable to have intercourse. It has at times been hard to trust that she is doing everything she can to fix the problem, because even though she works very hard now, there was a period when she ignored it, even though she promised to work on it. Things seem to be improving though now that she is in sex therapy and seeing a physical therapist.

3. **Would you say you are bothered by it in any way?**

    I am not sure how to answer this. Yes, it greatly affects my life, but I do not hold it against her.

4. **Does it make you depressed, angry or frustrated at times?**

    Yes, all of the above, though it's not directed towards her.

5. **Do you talk about the condition with her?**

    Yes, we often talk about it, around once per week.

6. **Have you ever sought out information on your own? If so, what was it and why?**

Yes, I have read extensively online about the condition and about treatment options, as well as read research papers on the subject. I read about it because I wanted to figure out if it was fixable, and if so then how to fix it. I know just about everything a layman can find out online about it.

7. **Do you help her with the dilators? Do you go with her to PT?**

Not yet, but the PT has recommended it.

8. **How do you help her with her condition?**

I talk about it, tell her about what I've read, encourage her, and help her to pay for therapy.

9. **What do you think or say when guys become angry at their partner for having this condition?**

I think it is immature for a guy to become angry at their partner for having the condition. I think it is understandable to become upset of their partner doesn't do anything about it.

10. **Does she often feel insecure or guilty with her condition? How do you help her then?**

Yes. I try to console her and tell her that I love her and will not leave her, and that I will help her through it however I can. I have gone to sex therapy with her before.

11. **Are you able to get intimate? This does not mean sex, but can be hand holding, cuddling, etc. If you can't, how does that make you feel?**

Yes, we are intimate in other ways than intercourse. I am a very physical person and require physical intimacy to feel loved.

12. **Does she also struggle with anxiety or depression?**

She struggles with generalized anxiety.

13. **What type of help is she receiving?**

She has seen a counselor for this and has tried medication, though she is not actively receiving help for it now. (Since she has left school things are less stressful.)

14. **Are you seeking help of any kind for yourself? (therapy, forums, etc.?)**

I just read.

15. **When did she tell you she had this condition?**

I think I knew before she did. A few years ago, she told me that she went in to get her first pap smear and it was too painful for them to do it. After googling, I was pretty sure she had it. It wasn't until we tried to have sex that it became clear. She saw a sex therapist who diagnosed her shortly after.

16. **How did you respond?**

I have tried to stay positive and respond optimistically.

~Anonymous

Duncan's Story

1. **What type of pelvic pain condition does your partner have?**

Vaginismus

2. **Does it affect your relationship? If so, how?**

Not from my perspective. I don't think it affects our relationship, but it bothers my partner. It affects her emotionally, which is then a problem. It's a problem because then she feels inadequate.

3. **Would you say you are bothered by it in any way?**

The lack of intimacy affects me because I would like to have that with my partner, but that lack of intimacy could be indirectly correlated with the vaginismus.

4. **Does it make you depressed, angry or frustrated at times**?

Emotional disturbance that my partner feels affects me. When she is hurt, I feel hurt. I don't feel depressed by the lack of intimacy, but it does make me feel sad at times because I want to be close to my partner.

5. **Do you talk about the condition with her?**

Yes, often.

6. **Have you ever sought out information on your own? If so, what was it and why?**

Yep, multiple books and online articles. I did it so that I could better understand it.

7. **Do you help her with the dilators? Do you go with her to PT?**

I've offered, and we plan to use the dilators together when she is ready.

8. **How do you help her with her condition?**

Being supportive and patient.

9. **What do you think or say when guys become angry at their partner for having this condition?**

Frustrated, it's like getting mad at someone for having a different eye color. It's not something that they can control.

10. **Does she often feel insecure or guilty with her condition? How do you help her then?**

    Yes, and I continue to be supportive and patient with her.

11. **Are you both able to get intimate? This does not mean sex, but can be hand holding, cuddling, etc. If you can't, how does that make you feel?**

    We can sometimes, but when we can't it's a little sad, but I will always be patient. It won't get better if I simply address it with anger.

12. **Does she also struggle with anxiety or depression?**

    Yes

13. **What type of help is she receiving?**

    Therapy, medication, dilators

14. **Are you seeking help of any kind for yourself? (therapy, forums, etc.?)**

    No

15. **When did she tell you she had this condition?**

    Before we dated

16. **How did you respond?**

    In a loving and supportive way. Trying to let her know that not every guy out there is the same and that she deserves to be treated with respect. ~ *Duncan, 25 (my fiancé)*

I was overwhelmed by how many men were eager to share their perspective on their partner's condition! So many came forward to volunteer and, in fact, more men came forward than women. Perhaps, this is because society has made it difficult for women to come forward to discuss their condition?

However, I did find it surprising that not every man knew what their partner's condition was and were able to correctly identify it by name. Only a handful sought help through therapy or forums but did take time to communicate with their partner about their condition. One thing that was predominantly discussed through each partner was that their women all struggled with some form of anxiety and/or depression.

Vaginismus is caused by anxiety and depression is often attributed to vaginismus later on, due to the dejected feelings the women develop. The majority of men all agreed that they try to be as supportive as possible with their significant other, and that it is frustrating at times but not worth getting angry over. Despite one exception, most stated that they would rather help their partner work through the problem than simply end the relationship and consider everything a lost cause.

Chapter 13: How do I cope?

This was a tough question for me to answer, and one that was recently asked via email. I had never been asked this question before or anything similar to it. It really caught me off guard.

I had to think long and hard before I could reply to this person because I didn't want to give them a false perspective on vaginismus and say that "It's all about staying positive!" because, truthfully, that's almost impossible.

How do I cope? This question was swimming in my mind for a full day and night until finally I just said to myself, "I simply have to be honest, even if it's not some enlightening response. I don't want to sugarcoat it for her."

My response was:

"I'm so glad you found this blog and contacted me! I'll be honest, when I first got this message, I wasn't sure how to respond. I had never been asked this question before and I kept thinking to myself, "how do I cope?"

In all honesty, this isn't an easy question for me to answer. Most days, I don't cope very well. I don't want to give you some bullshit response, like "be positive," because I feel like I would be lying to you when, in reality, I'm struggling with it all the time.

I wracked my brain for the right words to say to you and, honestly, the best advice that I can give is that you must take it one day at a time. It's so important to have a support group with you as well, whether that is a friend, a family member, a significant other or a therapist. Just let them be there for you so that you can vent and express yourself to them. Even if I turn out to be that person, please feel free to contact me. It's much better for your body and mind to vent than to let your depression and rage fester.

I know there are going to be a lot of hard days ahead of you, and I know that some days are going to be harder than the others. However, you just have to keep reminding yourself that you are a strong woman and that you can conquer anything. Breathing techniques, yoga, walking, exercises and stretches that my physical therapist gave me (which I'll provide in a blog soon), are helpful to ease the mind when you're all over the place. The stretches and breathing are also good for the PC muscles. Maybe even light a candle or create a calming place for yourself to meditate or breathe.

I would also recommend finding a hobby to keep your mind off the vaginismus and worrying about it. Nevertheless, this does not mean that you should pretend the condition doesn't exist. If you haven't yet, make sure you see a gynecologist, doctor, a physical therapist, or maybe even a therapist, so that you can get help and treatment for it. Who knows, there may even be treatment out there that works for you but doesn't work for me?

It's best to try different treatment options that are out there because you never know what ones may work for you. You might even be fortunate to live in a bigger city, where there are more options out there for you. I live in a small town, where the doctors aren't that great, and we don't have a lot of good physical therapists.

I don't want you to feel discouraged after reading this or think that you're only ever going to have bad days. Even if it doesn't seem like it right now, you're going to get through it. You're a strong woman and a strong individual. I'd be lying if I said it isn't hard, but you have to be a very strong person to deal with something like this. If you ever find yourself faltering and your emotions become too much, simply go to your support person and tell them how you are feeling. Tell them that you are struggling and need someone to talk to, even if it's just a shoulder to cry on.

I truly hope this helped and answered your question of how I deal with it. I'm going to post more blogs soon about exposure therapy and the stretches I was given by my physical therapist. These might really benefit you, so stay updated."

That was not only honest, but probably the longest email I had ever written. Hopefully, she didn't just take one look at it and toss it because of all the text

Regardless, I hope this helped someone else who is struggling with coping. It is a hard condition to fight through and it's not easy to live with mentally and emotionally.

Whoever you are out there that sent me this email, just stay strong and find that support.

Chapter 14: Don't Forget to Reward Yourself

It can be difficult to find ways to distract yourself when you become extremely depressed with vaginismus. Blogging helped me, but I also don't want to forget to explain how important it is to reward yourself from time to time, especially when things become physically and emotionally draining or demanding. My therapist was the one who brought this idea to me, because I was constantly feeling guilty about not using my dilators daily. She asked me what sounds more realistic for me to accomplish in a day or a week.

At first, I thought using the dilators at least twice a week was possible, as long as I made a schedule to use them. She said that I need to make sure I reward myself after using them.

It doesn't have to be extravagant or expensive. It can be as simple as watching your favorite movie in bed, lighting a candle, having time to yourself or even going out and buying a new candle (she knows I am obsessed with candles.)

Chapter 15: Viagra vs. Vaginismus

A little bit of a rant here...I simply can't wrap my head around the fact that research can be done to help men with erectile dysfunction, but they can't do more research to help women with painful vaginas.

Actually, I can wrap by head around it. Not to get all political, but I think society is downplaying some women's issues. Research has shown that 43 percent of women and 31 percent of men suffer from sexual dysfunctions.[11] A CNN article emphasized that "when Viagra hit the market, it changed the face of sexuality for men." However, research on female sexual dysfunction was and is still "significantly lagging."[12]

I mean, I'm not saying research should just stop for men who have erectile dysfunction, because that is a serious problem that

---

[11] Sexual Dysfunction," Cleveland Clinic, "2018, np.
[12] KFOR-TV, L. Noland and CNN Wire, "Where's my orgasm? Health experts target sexual dysfunction," Oklahoma's News, August 2018, np.

many men struggle with and it affects them emotionally and mentally, but vaginismus affects women the same way.

I just wish a little more research would be put out there for us as well. It seems kind of double standards for society to be okay talking about men's problems, but they view it as being taboo when women bring up their issues.

There are vast amounts of assistance for men with sexual dysfunction and very little out there for women's sexual dysfunction. Why is that okay? We struggle just as much as they do?

Chapter 16: Sex sells, but it doesn't have to…

We all love differently. For example, some of us are extremely affectionate, while others are not. There is nothing wrong with either of those traits. You are who you are, and you shouldn't be forced to change your personality just because your partner doesn't like it.

I am not affectionate by nature. When people give me hugs, I feel extremely awkward. I cannot kiss in public without feeling like everyone is watching me. I often need my space from my partner because that's just who I am. I am not aware of how little I give my partner kisses or hugs but, to me, I see what I'm doing as extremely normal. I'm not trying to be less affectionate and I certainly love my fiancé unconditionally, but I don't express it in the same way that he does.

If you are in a relationship with someone who is affectionate and perhaps you are not, or even vice versa, that's not a terrible thing. Every relationship has something that they need to work on. A relationship is two different people, who were raised differently and have different backgrounds, coming together to create their own family. Obviously, you are not always going to agree. It's important to communicate to your partner how he/she feels.

When they say communication is key, they truly mean it. It's vital to sit down with your partner and discover what they want and how they feel. Since I am not affectionate by nature, but my fiancé is, I would ask him what he feels deprived in. With the added layer of guilt from the vaginismus, I feel like an awful person for depriving him of both sex, intimacy and affection. However, by asking and communicating my feelings to him, I can learn to understand his needs more clearly. Together, we can come up with new ways to feel deeply connected and express affection. Metaphorically, since we are both different in that way, we need to build a road that both of us feel comfortable walking down together.

Despite what society is making us believe, we do not need to feel deeply connected through sex. This is also truly important to express to women who have vaginismus. You can be deeply connected with a person in so many other ways. This can be as simple as holding your partners hand or arm and truly being present and in that moment. This can also be just holding their face in your hand or outlining their face as you gaze into their eyes. You can also feel deeply connected by simply massaging each other.

You don't even need to use touch to be deeply connected if you struggle with affection. You can go on a trip together, explore new areas, cook with one another, watch a movie or even find passion in any adventure. You can also try to think back to when the two of you first started dating. What were some of the cute things you would do or say to one another in the beginning? For instance, my fiancé and I used to leave each other little love letters or notes. We haven't done that in years, but we are going to start up again because it's fun, yet still affectionate enough for him and not too demanding for my less affectionate nature.

At first, for those of you who don't struggle with sexual dysfunction, doing these things may seem silly because you are so used to using sex to express a deep connection. For those of us who can't have sex, or are just naturally less affectionate, we find alternatives that are just as rewarding. Maybe even more.

I think it's important for people to understand that sex isn't everything. The media, TV, movies, music and even our peers (thanks to society), have our heads spinning with images and fallacies that sex is crucial to every relationship, when in truth, there are many other ways to feel a deep connection with someone.

It makes me so sad that society has warped the minds of so many individuals, including kids, that sex is how a relationship is formed and how you keep it lasting. Society is obsessed with sex. It puts sex on a giant pedestal, as though it is the only thing that matters in a relationship.

You see sex everywhere. It's not like you can escape it. You see it on billboards, tabloids, magazines, in the mall, walking through a grocery store, etc.

As an experiment, I want you to just walk around your city and see how many times you spot something sexual. It is mind blowing but, I suppose, sex sells.

Chapter 17: Why can't we talk about sex?

Why can't we talk about sex? Why is it taboo? Why is it taboo when the media is obsessed with sex?

I find it so frustrating that talking about sexual dysfunctions, especially for females, is not something that is socially acceptable. Why do people have a hard time discussing sex and sexual problems? Meanwhile, sex is literally everywhere in our culture.

We are receiving mixed messages from our society about sex. Do we talk about it or is it not acceptable? If we don't talk about sex, then we become ignorant on the subject and on specific issues that relate to sex...like vaginismus and other sexual conditions.

Sex is not a big deal, yet people make it a big deal. It's a natural thing, but some people pretend it doesn't exist. I went to a Catholic school for seventeen years and having sex was not talked about. Literally, all they discussed was abstinence. How does that help?

People get very excited about pregnancy and babies, but refuse to talk about sex. They refuse to teach teenagers how to have safe sex and discuss the risks and challenges that can occur if you have it. They DO realize how those babies are made, right?

Having been told over and over and over again that sex is dirty, sex is bad, sex is sinful, warped my undeveloped brain. I believed all of this was true and, guess what, it not only warped by brain, but it also warped my PC muscles. They went into full defense mode. If sex is bad, then clearly, we (the PC muscles) should protect our person from having it ever.

Having vaginismus for eight years now, my muscles simply can't be told to relax. They don't even remember how to relax anymore. They have to relearn how to relax and this is not an easy process. I mean, I'm still working on it and it's been eight years. Thanks everyone. Thanks brain. Thanks PC muscles.

I get that many people view sex as something that is precious and only meant for husband and wife. I totally respect that. It truly is precious, and I believe that you should only have sex with someone who truly respects you and that you love unconditionally. However, for me, this does not mean only after marriage.

I grew up in a Catholic household and sex was never spoken about. We simply avoided the topic. I remember sitting on the kitchen counter one day on college break, trying to discuss sex with my mom, but she kept walking away to do laundry. I just gave up. I was deeply confused and merely wanted to ask her why sex was so painful and if that was common.

I'm not a parent though, so I can't judge. But I truly needed her, just like I need her now.

Just once, I would love to have a conversation about vaginismus and sex without the awkwardness. In fact, I would like to have a conversation about it period. I would love that to happen to everyone!

It kills me inside that family can joke about sex, but we can't have a serious discussion about a sexual problem. Especially, a sexual problem that is killing me emotionally. I mean, it's caused me to become medicated for goodness sake.

I cried to my fiancé about how I feel like no one cares because no one wants to discuss it. I often feel so alone with this problem, but I don't want any one of you to feel the same way.

Chapter 18: A Vaginismus Honeymoon

Weddings are exciting! They are magical, and something that every girl has dreamt of since she was able to walk around in her mom's high heels and dance around in a pillow case...That may or may not have happened...

I am so thrilled to get married. By the end of the first week of being engaged, I already had my dress, made the guest list, picked out my flowers and colors, picked a theme and made a music playlist. By week two, we had a venue and caterer.

Yeah, I know...it's a bit scary, but I hate procrastinating.

Needless to say, a lot of the big parts of the wedding were planned early, but I can't help to become nervous and terrified about the honeymoon portion.

We have already decided to spend it in Chicago, but I'm terrified it'll end up like our Valentine's trip to Chicago, where we were unable to get intimate and I spent the whole night crying with a bottle of wine.

My friends and I would envision and joke about our honeymoons being as spectacular and romantic as the movies.

But will mine? Or will it be a massive disappointment because of my condition?

This question keeps looming over me, making me distressed to work on wedding stuff at all.

For two months, I was on the ball, ready to plan and prepare for any wedding project or dilemma that appeared. After that surge now I am just tired. I am stressed, anxious, depressed, emotional and concerned because I want it to be magical and, right now, my fiancé and I haven't been able to get intimate or have sex in what - a year and a half or two years? You stop keeping track because it becomes depressing after a while. Lately, I've even cried watching the honeymoon scene on *Breaking Dawn*. Yeah, I know. I've reached a new level of low.

In all seriousness, all I want is a real honeymoon with my fiancé and a beautiful future with him.

Chapter 19: Vaginismus and Pregnancy

So one day, I received a bizarre letter in the mail. It was a letter inviting me to join a new mother's club. Either they know something I don't or there was clearly a mistake somewhere.

I'm not entirely sure why I received this, and it definitely had me chuckling a bit, but then got me thinking, which is sometimes a good thing…

One question that has always been on my mind is whether or not having a baby while you have vaginismus will work out. In fact, the third most common question I get asked when someone finds out that I have vaginismus is "So, can you have kids?"

To be honest, there is a part of me that isn't sure I want to have kids because I have such bad anxiety. Then, there is another part of me that kind of wants them.

Nevertheless, I did my research on this topic and thought I'd share my insights with those of you who are wondering the exact same thing. This is a common concern with women who have vaginismus and consider planning a family with children. Will they be able to get pregnant? How will the pregnancy go? What about examinations? What about the birth? What will happen with the vaginismus and the muscles after giving birth?

All of these are great and important questions that we will explore now.

1.) Can I get pregnant?

Yes. You are able to get pregnant if you are able to have sex with your partner or, if not, through self- insemination. Dr. Pacik stated in his blog, Pregnancy and Vaginismus, on the Maze Women's Sexual Health website that some patients with vaginismus conceived a child and were still virgins! No, they were not impregnated by the Holy Spirit. Instead, their partners could "do the deed," so to speak, by the genital lips leading up to prime ovulation period, and still became pregnant. Crazy! However, if you are having difficulties getting pregnant, seek a doctor's advice.[13]

2.) **What will the pregnancy be like?**

Typically, like every other pregnancy. The pelvic examination and vaginal ultrasound may be extremely difficult for a woman with vaginismus. Some doctors might even have to work on the outside of the woman's vagina to see what's going on with baby; however, this adds a whole new level of risk if the doctor can't feel what's happening on the inside.[14]

3.) **What will childbirth be like?**

Well, some doctors will tell their patient, who has vaginismus, that a C-section is the best route for them. However, a C-section is not a must. The pelvic floor muscles open up naturally during childbirth, making it possible for women with vaginismus to give birth naturally.[15]

---

[13] Peter T. Pacik, "Pregnancy and Vaginismus," Maze Women's Sexual Health, April 2018, np.

[14] "Vaginismus, pregnancy and childbirth," Women's Therapy Center, November 16, 2017, np.

[15] Lbid.

4.) Now that I have had the baby, what will my vaginal muscles be like?

As Dr. Pacik stated in his blog, unless those initial fears, triggers and anxieties were fixed prior, during or after the baby was born, you will likely still have vaginismus. [16]

While there are stories of women undergoing vaginal childbirth and discovering their vaginismus was gone, there are just as many who discovered that it worsened. Unfortunately, it's a risk you must take if you plan to give birth vaginally while you have vaginismus.

Chapter 20: How and when to tell your partner that you have Vaginismus or Pelvic Pain

I have come across numerous posts and emails from women regarding when and how they should tell the person that they are dating about vaginismus.

This is a fantastic question, and one I often thought about myself when I was dating. At first, because I just wanted to narrow down my options, I told the guys right up front that this is the condition I have and, basically, you can either stay or go (of course I worded it in a much nicer way than that). However, the responses I would receive were often:

"Don't worry, I can fix you."

"I'm sure I'll be able to help you to get over it."

---

[16] Lbid.

"Wait? Are you serious or just trying to get me away from you?"

"Wow, you must be cursed!"

"Oh…"

…or they simply just laughed and/or stopped texting me altogether.

I truly hope that none of you run into a person who refuses to listen, and instead, tries to force you to do other things, as if you owe them something. That's a situation no one should be in.

All of those responses were either rude or extremely cocky and, in the end, none of them could handle the situation. From my experience, it generally takes 3-4 months for a guy who says, "I can fix you," to give up and leave.

So, my words of advice (take it or leave it) are to approach each relationship with caution. Really learn who they are and what their intentions are in the relationship. Build trust with them and, finally, when you are truly comfortable with this person, explain the situation to them. Their words and actions should give you your answer.

However, sometimes, the truth has to come out sooner than you expected. Explain the condition to him as best as you can. If he is a decent guy and willing to be there to support you and talk about the condition with you, then relax. Those whose intentions are good will ask questions, listen to you and research topics relating to vaginismus with you or on his own time. He will hold you during the difficult days and gently coax you to not give up during the days that you want to.

It takes a very strong and patient individual to go through this with someone and, even then, the most patient person can crack at times. It's human nature. Just talk about it. Communication is so important, especially when there is no physical intimacy. Don't feel like a failure if you both need to go into therapy together. Personally, I think marriage counseling is great for every marriage, even if things are fine.

Also, remember that you are expecting a level of trust from him, so you should give that same level of trust back. By telling him about your condition, you are being truly honest with him. I know it might be scary at first, especially if you truly care for this person and are afraid you might lose him, but if his response is not appropriate then you just saved yourself a lot of heartbreak and tears down the line.

It's better to have those high standards and know when to walk away from someone than to stay because you love them and, later on, have their words and actions negatively affect your vaginismus even more.

Chapter 21: How does vaginismus affect your partner?

One day, as I'm lying in bed with a hurt back (my dog had been getting cold outside, so I picked him up immediately to be carried inside and, apparently, 50 pounds is too much for me), I stumbled upon a Free Sex Podcast on SoundCloud about vaginismus called *#39 Vaginismus: We Can't Have Sex*.

In the podcast episode, they discuss various treatments, how vaginismus can affect you and your partner, how it's a widely avoided topic, and how this can happen to anyone of any age.

The main takeaway I had from listening to their conversation is that I am extremely glad that they discussed how your partner might feel and what they can do to alleviate some of the stress. For me, I always feel guilty because I know it's difficult for him and that it can cause any man to feel insecure in a relationship. However, instead of feeling this guilt, I should be productive and do something to show him that I am still attracted to him, even if intimacy and affection are difficult for me. This lack of affection makes dealing with vaginismus so much worse for him emotionally. Again, I'm feeling the guilt as he is silently sleeping next to me, unknowingly inching closer to me in his slumber.

Katie and Candice mentioned that there should be a support group for men, and I 100% agree, because it is an extremely difficult thing for partners to go through and understand. Many men might feel hurt or rejected, they might feel inadequate or even become depressed by the lack of intimacy. It's important for the couples to talk about how they feel and discuss what their wants and needs are because, let's face it, vaginismus can negatively impact a relationship easily.

Because this lack of intimacy and the lack of sex can take years to overcome, it can cause severe strain on the relationship. I know firsthand that it can. I won't lie, it's hard. It's hard for me and it's hard for my fiancé. We have had numerous arguments (although he would call them discussions) about the lack of intimacy. Therefore, communication is key, and so is listening to what your partner has to say about how he is feeling. When couples bottle up their emotions, which I have been guilty of doing, it only leads to frustration and anger. If men bottle up their true feelings about how vaginismus affects them, simply because they are worried how it might affect their partner's feelings, then those pent-up emotions can lead to depression and, later on, resentment.

It really does make me smile that this podcast is out there, helping women and men who are looking for advice. They mentioned that vaginas have been negatively viewed over the years as taboo or a mystery that girls shouldn't touch or talk about. Nevertheless, it is considered normal for boys to discover masturbating at a young age, while girls are often taught the exact opposite. The podcast recommended that women should spend a few minutes every day looking at their vaginas in a mirror to take away that anxiety or shame we might feel.

Chapter 22: Eliminate the shame of sex for women

So how do you find a good physical therapist and how many women have a hard time not viewing their vaginas as dirty because of beliefs they were taught early in life?

On the episode, *How To: Heal Vaginal Pain During Sex (Vaginismus)*, of the Free Sex Podcast, they had a certified Physical Therapist from Pennsylvania, Ashlie Crewe, join them to discuss the topic of vaginismus.

Ashlie reiterated that vaginismus is like a panic attack of the pelvic floor muscles that can be brought on from anything, even UTIs or Yeast Infections. She stated that studies were done that showed how women with yeast infections or UTIs were unable to get rid of the inflammation in their vaginal walls after having these illnesses. Basically, their vaginas were never able to go back to the way they once were before these infections occurred.

Ashlie also stated that many Christian religions teach women, from a young age, that sex is dirty or should be experienced only after marriage. These girls are taught to not touch or talk about their vaginas, yet once they are older and get married, they are expected to become sexual beings with their husbands. Ashlie, Katie and Candice emphasized that this is not a healthy way to go about teaching sex to young girls.

Ashlie had a patient, who was brought up Catholic, and was told over and over again that sex is supposed to hurt for women, especially if you are a good girl. How terrible that this poor woman went years with the belief that painful sex was the norm! She didn't even tell her gynecologist because she thought every woman was dealing with this.

Instead of sex shaming these girls at a young age, we should be supportive and provide good parental advice on the topic. Exploring the body when you are little shouldn't be shameful, as long as it's done in a private location. I was terrified to touch or even look at my genitals growing up because of the church teachings that I was taught, and I often wonder who I would have been if they hadn't been so strict on us girls.

Parents should be realistic and tell their children that they will love and support them even if they mess up. A healthy, balanced approach with this topic is so important, especially in today's society. Make sure that your daughter knows you will always be there for her. Don't have your fears of her having sex at all cause her to get vaginismus later in life.

Delving into the physical therapy aspect of this discussion, Ashlie stated that traditional therapy should be incorporated with your physical therapist. A good physical therapist should also massage your muscles during each session to find any triggers in the muscles and to help release tension in the pelvic floor region.

She even talked about how women, who are working on having sex with their partners, should understand that the pain is much worse during penetration. She advised that women should perform diaphragmatic breathing during sex to help ease tension in the nervous system.

She said that if the pain becomes too much during the act, simply tell your significant other to stop moving but don't pull out, because pulling out will only cause the muscles to clamp shut again. When the man responds to this, it lets the woman know she has control of the situation, which will put her at ease and help her to relax.

Ashlie also recommended that, for the first couple of times, the woman should be on top, because this allows her to go at her own pace and stop to breathe whenever she needs to.

Chapter 23: Don't hide from the condition...

It's hard to admit that something is wrong with your body or even your mind. It took me a long time to admit that I had vaginismus. Reading about it online, prior to being officially

110

diagnosed, was horrifying to say the least. I couldn't comprehend how a trigger, that I couldn't even discern, was causing my body to be in physical pain. I would think to myself, "How is this a real thing and how can it possibly be fixed?"

Unfortunately, because of my fears of telling others and the fears (and me) being seen as abnormal, I kept it a secret for so long and just felt lost and hopeless. I wept at the realization that I couldn't do something that everyone around me was enjoying. I felt alone, not only because I didn't know anyone around me who suffered from the same condition, but also because I couldn't express the pain that I was going through. It wasn't until my therapist helped me to come to terms with this emotional struggle that I finally sought out real medical attention.

I know that there are many women out there who are also struggling to admit that they have vaginismus. I completely understand, and I can truly sympathize. It's extremely difficult to admit that you can't have sex. However, I promise, that once you talk to someone about it and seek medical help, you will feel relief. I know you might be thinking, "Well, once I talk to a doctor, what can they actually do for me? How long will I have this? Will I ever be able to have sex?"

The answer is yes; you will be able to have sex again. The journey for vaginismus varies for everyone. What might take years for one women, might only be months for another. Treatments for vaginismus vary for each woman as well. One treatment might work for Jane, but that same one might not work for Ann. Ann must then talk to her doctor or research another treatment.

Just because something doesn't work out for you doesn't mean that you should give up hope. I lost hope when I was turned away by countless doctors and gynecologists. I lost hope when every treatment I knew of at the time failed to work on me. I lost hope for almost a year, until I started my blog. Now, as I'm reaching out to others and acquiring connections with women, who struggle with this condition and who have overcome it, I feel that there is hope after all.

Some of you might even avoid going to an examination because you are terrified of the pain. I totally get that. I hate going to examinations because I become anxious, tense and cry without even realizing it. One time, my heart rate was so high during an examination, that they had me perform breathing exercises right there on the examination table. More than one nurse always has to be present in the room because I can't stop shaking due to the pain. Sometimes, they will even have a nurse hold my hand and talk to me while the examination is occurring. It does make me feel abnormal, but in all reality, it truly shouldn't. This is just who I am at the moment, but I will continue to be strong and persevere.

Despite the anxiety you might feel entering the doctor's office, it is important to go see one, especially if you aren't sure that you have the condition. Finding out what is going on with your body will allow the doctor to help you as best as they can.

What I'm trying to say is that you shouldn't be scared to seek help. We all need a little help sometimes and finding support for vaginismus is a crucial step to overcoming it. Don't worry about what people might think of you or what society is telling you. They don't matter anyways. Instead, focus on you. Focus on relaxing and helping yourself conquer this condition that I bet many people wouldn't even be able to deal with. You are enough, and you are stronger than you think.

Resources for You

If you are looking for more information on Pelvic Support, Amy Stein and Ashlie Crew gave a few resources such as, the International Pelvic Pain Society and the National Vulvodynia Association. For physical therapists, both suggested visiting the Herman and Wallace Institute, as well as the American Physical Therapy Association. I'll list some of these that they mentioned below:

International Pelvic Pain Society
– https://www.pelvicpain.org/home.aspx
Beyond Basics Physical Therapy Practice
– http://www.beyondbasicsphysicaltherapy.com
Heal Pelvic Pain Book – http://www.healpelvicpain.com/
National Vulvodynia Association – https://www.nva.org/
Interstitial Cystitis Association – https://www.ichelp.org/
Herman & Wallace – https://hermanwallace.com/
American Physical Therapy Association – https://www.apta.org/

Bibliography

Carter, Mark and Lisa. *Completely Overcome Vaginismus: The Practical Approach to Pain-Free Intercourse.* 2011.

Diagnostic and Statistical Manual of Mental Disorders. American Psychiatric Association. 5th ed. 2013.

Harvey-Jenny, Catriona. "I had to have botox in my vagina so I could lose my virginity." Cosmopolitan. April 10, 2017. https://www.cosmopolitan.com/uk/love-sex/sex/a9255298/vaginismus-treatment-botox-success/.

KFOR-TV, L. Noland and CNN Wire. "Where's my orgasm? Health experts target sexual dysfunction." Oklahoma's News. August 2018. https://kfor.com/2014/08/08/wheres-my-orgasm-health-experts-target-sexual-dysfunction/.

Lytle, Devin. "I Got Botox In My Vagina And It Changed My Life." BuzzFeed. January 13, 2017. https://www.buzzfeed.com/laraparker/i-got-botox-in-my-vagina-and-it-changed-my-life?utm_term=.hgXZ0mRQr#.qg7RDMLOz.

Merriam-Webster Dictionary online, *"courage,"* 2018. https://www.merriam-webster.com/dictionary/courage.

Pacik, Peter T. "Botox Injection for Treatment of Vaginismus." U.S. National Library of Medicine. 2017. https://clinicaltrials.gov/ct2/show/NCT01352546.

Pacik, Peter T. *How, Why and How Often is Botox Used to Treat Vaginismus?* Vaginismus MD. 2018. https://www.vaginismusmd.com/vaginismus-treatment-dr-peter-pacik/botox-treatment/how-botox-works/.

Pacik, Peter T. "Pregnancy and Vaginismus." Maze Women's Sexual Health. April 2018. https://www.mazewomenshealth.com/blog/2016/12/01/pregnancy-and-vaginismus/.

Pacik, Peter T. *Understanding and treating vaginismus: a multimodal approach.* The International Urogynecology Association. 2014.

"Sexual Dysfunction." Cleveland Clinic. 2018. https://my.clevelandclinic.org/health/diseases/9121-sexual-dysfunction.

"Vaginismus, pregnancy and childbirth." Women's Therapy Center. Nov. 16, 2017. http://www.womentc.com/blog/vaginismus-pregnancy-childbirth/.

Werner MA, Pacik PT, Ferrara M, Marcus BS. *Botox for the Treatment of Vaginismus: A Case Report.* Journal of Women's Health Care. 2014. https://www.omicsonline.org/open-access/botox-for-the-treatment-of-vaginismus-a-case-report-2167-0420.1000150.php?aid=24905.

"What is Neurofeedback?" OchsLabs: The Neurofeedback Experts. 2018. https://www.site.ochslabs.com/about.

Made in the USA
Middletown, DE
21 April 2019